BREATHE LIKE A BADASS

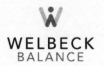

WELBECK
BALANCE

About the Author

Hannah Jane Thompson is a qualified meditation and mindfulness teacher, and certified life coach, whose training is in mindfulness-based cognitive therapy (MBCT), and the principles of Theravada Buddhism.

She runs Breathe Like A Badass, an online personalized meditation service helping ambitious-but-anxious women all over the world beat stress and anxiety, calm their inner critic, do more of what they love without burnout – and actually enjoy life.

Hannah discovered meditation herself over a decade ago, after years of struggling with anxiety, low self-worth, bad breakups, lack of career direction, and even less self-compassion or self-belief. It saved her life, and now she helps others discover it too.

BREATHE LIKE A BADASS

Beat Anxiety & Self-Doubt, Calm Your Inner Critic & Build a
No-Nonsense Mindfulness & Meditation Toolkit

by Hannah Jane Thompson

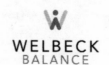

WELBECK
BALANCE

A Trigger Book
Published by Welbeck Balance
An imprint of Welbeck Publishing Group
20 Mortimer Street
London W1T 3JW

First published by Welbeck Balance in 2021

A CIP catalogue record for this book is available from the British Library

ISBN
Trade Paperback – 978-1-78956-288-0

Typeset by Lapiz Digital Services
Printed in Great Britain by CPI Group (UK) Ltd, Croydon CR0 4YY

10 9 8 7 6 5 4 3 2 1

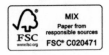

Note/Disclaimer

Welbeck Balance encourages diversity and different viewpoints. However, all views,
thoughts, and opinions expressed in this book are the author's own and are not
necessarily representative of Welbeck Publishing Group as an organization. All
material in this book is set out in good faith for general guidance; no liability can
be accepted for loss or expense incurred in following the information given. The
author of this book has sought to be as inclusive and sensitive as possible to people
of all experiences, abilities, faiths, genders, sexualities, ethnicities, backgrounds
and beliefs. In particular, this book is not intended to replace expert medical or
psychiatric advice. It is intended for informational purposes only and for your own
personal use and guidance. It is not intended to diagnose, treat or act as a substitute
for professional medical advice. Meditation can work as a complement to therapy
and mental health treatment plans, but not as a replacement for them. Those with
severe mental health issues should approach meditation with caution; and if needed,
only under the supervision of a professional. The author is not a medical practitioner
nor a licensed therapist and professional advice should be sought if desired before
embarking on any health-related programme.

www.welbeckpublishing.com

To Oli, my rainbow in every storm.
To my parents, who always pick up the phone.

And to everyone brave enough to sit with ourselves, look inward and choose compassion. We are all badasses.

Contents

Introduction

What Does "Breathe Like A Badass" Even Mean?

"You can be in a huge crowd, but if you don't feel like you can trust anyone or talk to anybody, you feel like you're really alone."

Fiona Apple, singer-songwriter

It is bizarre that I am writing a book with the word "badass" in the title because, for most of my life, I have not felt remotely badass. Ten years ago, I wouldn't have even known what it meant.

I was what I would call an "ambitious-but-anxious" woman. I was a journalist working 9-to-5 in a central London office, with loads of qualifications, supportive parents, and what looked like a great life. But I was slowly suffocating under inexplicable sadness, anxiety, depression, and what I felt was shameful misery; with a negative and bitchy inner critic running the show, and a feeling that my life was happening somewhere else without me.

I knew I had potential, and had always worked hard. I knew I wanted a happy, big, juicy, successful life. I knew I wanted my career to be meaningful. I knew there had to be more to existence than feeling totally stuck in my job – unproductive, unfulfilled, numb, constantly second-guessing myself and feeling miserable

AF – but I didn't know how to even begin to calm the swirling anxiety inside my mind. I'd worked for years for the life I had. I told myself this was just "how it was" – I just needed to cope better. And I was utterly ashamed for having such a privileged life, and still hating it.

Growing up, I'd believed that when things get tough, you should get tougher. Try harder. Sleep less. "Get your shit together!", my brain shouted at me a thousand times a day. Like so many ambitious, high-achieving people, throughout my life I'd believed that if I was harsher to myself – stayed at my desk a little longer, forced myself to keep going, ignored my feelings, suppressed the real me, and tried to mould myself into who I thought I "should be" – or who someone else told me I "should be" – that somehow, I'd succeed... whatever that meant.

So I stayed small, stuck, jealous, bitter, anxious, scared, full of self-doubt and pain and excuses, getting nowhere fast. And when it got really bad, I thought I should just have a G&T or some chocolate, have a laugh, and lighten up. After all, we can't all be happy, all the time, can we? That was it. That was the extent of my emotional education. And it worked – until it didn't.

A life problem

I never had a drinking problem. But I *did* have a life problem. Depression, anxiety, panic, zero ability to cope with anything. I cried on trains, got stupid stuff wrong at work, isolated myself from friends, avoided mirrors in case I saw my own reflection, and fantasized about maybe accidentally-on-purpose getting hit by a London bus so I wouldn't have to live inside my own brain for a single day longer.

I woke up crying every day, and felt like I was failing at everything. I even developed this weird image of a terrifying black whirlpool in my head. I didn't know how to stop it. And I knew I was privileged. So I reckoned the problem had to be with me.

I vividly recall standing on the platform of the District Line at Victoria Underground Station, feeling the raised concrete dots beneath my feet, my eyes transfixed by the yellow MIND THE GAP writing at the edge of the platform, unable to muster the conviction to jump in front of the train. I was so devoid of compassion for myself that I didn't think I *deserved* to die. I was too boring, stupid, lazy and predictable for that. It would just annoy everyone, and I'd probably fuck it up anyway. Maybe that's a sign that I hadn't yet hit "rock bottom". But it felt pretty damn low to me.

And if any of that sounds remotely familiar – from low-level anxiety to full-blown depression – know this: *You're not alone, and there is hope.* I know there is, because on one random grey evening, I saw an article poking out from one of my then-flatmate's piles of magazines. As I remember it, the headline said: "Think yourself happy."

I was sceptical, but something sparked in my brain. I thought thinking too much was my problem. But this article said you could actually use thinking to help yourself. What? Doubtfully, I read the interview with this bald dude, a former Buddhist monk, about his little-known London-based meditation app and events company, Headspace. (Headspace is now a multimillion-dollar behemoth, with more than 65 million downloads. But it wasn't then.) The article changed my life. Maybe, just maybe, I didn't deserve to feel so utterly crap, and could question that negative inner voice. Maybe I could stop the swirling black whirlpool in my head. I learned I wasn't alone in feeling like this. The big questions I was struggling with had answers.

Not to be dramatic, but meditation saved my life. Of course, it wasn't instant. It took years of unravelling and unlearning, of trying again and again to be kinder to myself. The process is still happening. But through the principles of mindfulness and meditation, my life has transformed. I've learned to manage my feelings gently, to be aware of them without masking them, to find calm and focus even when anxiety and depression loom. I have rewired my brain so it no longer says, "I can't, I'm not good enough!" and instead asks, "Why *not* me?".

In so many ways, we are what we think. If we can change the way we think and react – from negative and critical to purposeful and positive – we can transform our own lives, breath by breath. This book is all about how helping you to do that – to build a life that feels transformative, purposeful and positive.

Fast-forward to now. I'm a certified mindfulness meditation teacher, and specialize in helping high-achieving, ambitious women – just like I was – to beat anxiety, stress and burnout. I work with them to calm their inner critic, balance work and rest, and build mindful success, so that they too can be successful and happy, whatever that means to them.

I now know that taking care of your mental and emotional health is the key to success, whether you're trying to start your own business – to go freelance or set up that side hustle – get promoted, leave a bad job or relationship, find a brilliant job or relationship, make more money than you believe possible, or simply want to wake up feeling a bit less shit and anxious – and happier and more confident in your own skin. And I'm here to help you do just that. I call this process "transforming your inner voice from bitch to badass", and I use the tools of mindfulness and meditation to form my main process. That's what I mean when I say "breathe like a badass". Because all we need in order to start using meditation effectively is our breath. It's free, it's simple and it's portable.

The tools of meditation have given me the emotional toolbox I needed in a world that often seems very scary and uncertain, and sometimes even impossible to survive. By remembering that – and through using those tools myself daily – I sometimes recognize in myself that inner badass I never even knew I had all those years ago.

Mind the perfection gap

There's just one caveat. I would never say, "All you need to do is follow the tools in this book, and you'll never have a single bad day again! I'm proof!" It doesn't work like that.

I still suffer from anxiety and comparison, and sometimes find myself scrolling through Instagram, comparing myself to seven thousand other people and wondering why it makes me feel like crap. I'm still hard on myself; I get caught in negativity spirals; I struggle with depression and anxiety; and I worry nothing I do is good enough. I'm not writing from a pedestal. Meditation is not magic, and nor are any other mental health tools you might discover. It's not a cure-all, a panacea to all of society's ills, and it doesn't "fix" everything. Don't believe anyone who says it does.

Long story short, I'm still my own worst critic. Perfection doesn't exist. So I won't promise it to you here. The difference is that I've learned how to question and quieten that inner critic, and, slowly but surely, change her from a bitch to a badass. I've learned how to master that negative inner voice, and turn it into something a little kinder and more helpful, instead.

It's my view that unhappiness is that gap between where we are and where we think we *should* be – and that gap can be massive. I've learned that no matter how your life looks from the outside, no matter what you achieve... if you still feel like shit on the inside... it's never going to be enough for you. No promotions, relationships, yoga classes, G&Ts, brunches, degrees, dates or sunny days will ever be enough if you don't address the negative inner critic in your own mind. And as you *have* to be inside your own head... why not try to make it a kinder, happier, nicer place to be?

It's no exaggeration to say that learning how to do that transformed my career and my business. Once I started fixing *the inside stuff*, the external stuff started getting better too. My business and freelance career went from strength to strength. I started taking opportunities I would never have noticed before. I now know how to remember that I'm good enough, no matter what, and everything else is a bloody great bonus.

Mindfulness and meditation taught me that the key to a successful, happy life isn't to beat yourself up mentally, or work longer hours, or try to force yourself to be or do something you hate. You don't need to prove yourself to others by working until you're completely exhausted, depressed, anxious and burned out. Learn to be kind to yourself, instead. Be your own best supporter. Rewire that inner critic into your coach. And that's why I'm so obsessed with meditation, and want you to be too.

That's what this book is about. Non-woo, zero-fluff, simple, totally doable, scientifically proven, human, practical, fit-it-into-your-life, get-it-done, approachable meditation. No chimes or chakras or chunks of rose quartz. If that's your bag, then great. But you won't find any of that stuff here. Because that's not what helped me. What helped me is basic, daily, breathe-in-breathe-out, don't-be-a-bitch-to-yourself, easy meditation.

At this point I should remind you that I'm not a doctor, Buddhist nun or trauma specialist. I have two degrees, but neither are in neuroscience. I'm not a replacement for a psychiatrist or a licensed psychologist, so if you feel that you need that kind of professional help, by all means please seek it out. But these techniques can, and do, work well alongside counselling or psychology. (In fact, many of my clients work with me and therapists at the same time.)

I am a certified meditation teacher and qualified life coach, who has worked with some great meditation teachers, counsellors and coaches. I take my responsibility as someone teaching meditation very seriously. I care about your mental health, and I know that when applied with care, persistence, patience and self-compassion, the techniques in this book can help.

I'm also a human who believes that every single person deserves to feel good about themselves and their life... even (especially!) you. That's why, since I discovered the power of meditation, I've been on a decade-long quest to discover the best, most scientifically proven ways out there to rewire your brain, and transform your inner voice from bitch to badass.

Because, if we set our minds to it, we can move motherfucking mountains. We can do great things, make good money, and feel a lot happier, too. To squander your potential, living a life wrapped up in self-doubt and unhappiness, feels like a tragic waste to me.

If you agree, you're in the right place. Breathe in, breathe out. Let's do this.

PART ONE

THE BASICS

1

Why Should I Meditate?

(or, What's In It for Me?)

"You can't stop the waves, but you can learn to surf."

Jon Kabat-Zinn, professor and mindfulness expert

Meditation is kind of a pain in the arse. I know – I'm a meditation teacher – I'm not supposed to say that. But it is. Because it's *always* easier *not* to do the thing than to do it! To stay on the sofa rather than go for a jog. To do what your parents and friends say, rather than trying something different or scary or new.

And it would be a lot easier for me to tell you that you could just take a pill to get all the benefits of meditation without having to find the time, energy, skills or patience to do it. Sadly, it doesn't work like that.

But that doesn't mean it's not worth doing. Here are some key benefits. This obviously isn't an exhaustive list, but I've cherry-picked a few that might be most relevant to you. Meditation has the power to:

- Boost self-compassion
- Calm anxiety, overthinking and depression
- Reduce stress and its physical symptoms
- Help you to manage heartbreak, disappointment and grief
- Heal or calm trauma
- Stop you comparing yourself to others
- Give you the courage to do what makes you happy (e.g., quit your dead-end job)
- Reduce stress, increase productivity and help you find your purpose
- Improve the quality of your sleep and rest
- Reduce phone addiction and help with digital detoxing
- Improve body image
- Increase your enjoyment of, and relationship with, food and alcohol
- Boost your enjoyment of movement, and improve your fitness and physical health
- Strengthen your relationships, communication and sex life
- Heal your relationship with money
- Build compassion for others, and your ability to address global issues

Each chapter of this book will take you through these benefits in turn. If any of the above sounds good to you, then meditation really can help.

How does it work?

Over the years, I've learned that when people ask *why* they should meditate, they actually mean *how*. They don't mean, "*How* do I do it?" (see the next chapter for that), but "How does it work? How, and why, does sitting down and focusing on my breathing achieve any one of these things? Sounds fake."

The short answer is: neuroplasticity. This is the concept that you can *literally change your brain*, even well into adulthood. You can physically rewire your brain to change the way you think, feel and react to situations, even after years of trauma, negative self-talk or learned habits. With neuroplasticity, you can take control of your brain, and change some bits you don't like or that aren't serving you anymore.

Our brain – and therefore what we think and how we act – is formed over the course of our lives. But at some point, many of us realize that our thoughts aren't exactly helpful, or kind. Or we find that we're so stressed, anxious or depressed that we feel on the point of imploding, and we've drunk enough gin to know the answer isn't in the bottle. So we look for answers. If we can change the way we *think*, then maybe we can change the way we behave and feel. And maybe, even if we can't totally change our thoughts overnight, it's just possible that we can change the way we *react* to them. That's what meditation helps us to do, gently and compassionately.

Meditating is for the brain what bicep curls are to the arms. As meditation teacher Jeff Warren writes in the book he co-authored with Dan Harris, *Meditation for Fidgety Skeptics*:

"Every time you catch yourself wandering and escort your attention back to the breath, it is like a bicep curl for the brain. It is also a radical act: you're breaking a lifetime's habit of walking around in a fog of rumination and projection, and you are actually focusing on what's happening right now."[1]

And just as doing a few bicep curls isn't going to get you instantly ripped, it's the same with meditation. It takes practice, consistency, faith, and doing a little bit often – rather than a single mammoth session once a month. That's because, just as you're building muscle at the gym, with meditation, you're building up – or changing the structure of – your brain. It takes time.

Imagine your brain as a road, and you're the driver of the car. The car is a thought or a habit. Following your usual patterns – negative self-talk or stress, say – is like speeding down the motorway. It's easier. It's already built for you, you know it, and it's the quickest route. Taking a different route would be like finding your way through darker back roads. It's harder. It takes more time. You'd have to do it deliberately, carefully and by changing your usual patterns. But, eventually, it will take you down a different, more scenic road that is more relaxing to drive down than a busy motorway. That's what we're doing with meditation.

Over time, you get to know the new route, and it becomes as easy as flying down the motorway... easier, even. But that takes time. It's ironic that I'm using a car metaphor, because I hate driving. But you get the picture.

René Descartes may have said: "I think, therefore I am," but the Buddhist nun Thubten Chodron wrote: "Don't believe everything you think."[2]

So when I say "rewire your brain", I mean it. And although meditation has been practised for thousands of years, and used to be known as a "spiritual, hippy" practice, modern science has started to prove that it *actually* works. Regular practice can make tangible, measurable, repeatable, visible changes in our brain – and therefore change our behaviour and feelings.

You can literally track it with a brain (fMRI) scan.[3] Mind-blowing, right? Very simply, meditation helps us strengthen the *prefrontal cortex*, the more-developed part of our brain that helps us respond in a more measured way to stressful situations. When we do this, we dampen down the *amygdala*, which is the more primitive "monkey" or "lizard" part of our brain, which has us *react* to things, rather than responding more rationally.

By changing our brain, we can train ourselves to *respond, not react*, to stressors. This means we can "step back" from our immediate actions or reactions, put a bit more space between us and our emotions and immediate knee-jerk actions, and choose a kinder, more peaceful, happier and less destructive road.

Studies show that the amygdala shows noticeably less reactivity after around 30 hours of mindfulness training over eight weeks. This is equivalent to 3.75 hours of meditation per week, or 32 minutes per day.[4] It's a commitment, sure, but not an unreasonable one. And you can start small at five or ten minutes a day, and work up.

Meditation: An adulting manual

Meditation doesn't only help rewire your brain and your habits for *you*. Studies also show that it can measurably improve your compassion for others.

And, they say, the results improve as you go.

In their incredible book, *The Science of Meditation: How to Change Your Brain, Mind and Body*, author and psychologist Daniel Goleman and neuroscientist and professor Richard J. Davidson, considered the brains of beginners (100 to 1,000 hours of meditation), "long-term" (9,000 hours+) and "yogi" Buddhist monk meditators (27,000 hours+), and concluded: "Sticking with meditation over the years offers more benefits... [and] practising meditation can pay off quickly... even if you have just started."[5]

This book is all about how and why the simple act of taking a few minutes a day to meditate, and continuing to persevere even when it's hard, is one of the most powerful things you can do for your mental and physical health. It's the only tool I've ever discovered that actually works in the long-term, and gives me (and my one-to-one clients, and millions of others learning from many other teachers) genuine lasting relief for anxiety, stress, fear, comparison, lack of self-worth, self-criticism and much more.

Not only that, but the Buddhist ethics and principles surrounding the act of meditation can also provide a framework for our lives – making us happier, healthier and less self-critical – even if we're not at all religious. If you've ever felt, like I have, that you need an instruction manual on how to "adult" in today's world, then meditation and its principles are the closest thing I've ever found to that.

2

Is Meditation Really for Me?

(or, These Meditation Myths are Holding you Back)

"If it weren't for my mind, my meditation would be excellent!"

Pema Chödrön, Buddhist nun

Whenever people find out I'm a meditation teacher, they usually say one of a few things. Be honest – how many of these have you thought or said before?

ATTITUDES TO MEDITATION QUIZ

Answer yes/no, and count up the number of yes answers.

1. I'm not the kind of person who meditates. Meditation is for other people, not me. Y/N
2. I'd love to meditate, but I'm too busy and never have enough time. Y/N

---

3. I am mindful in other ways, so I don't need to meditate. Y/N
4. I've tried it but was terrible at it, so I gave up. Y/N
5. Having a wellness routine is boring. I want to be spontaneous. Y/N
6. Meditation has been whitewashed and/or is only for rich people with more money than problems or sense. Y/N
7. Meditation makes you selfish and self-obsessed. Y/N
8. I can't just "live in the present" – I have shit to plan! Y/N
9. I'm afraid of what I'll find in my brain if I sit still and listen to my thoughts. Y/N

How many did you get?
1–3: Slightly sceptical
4–6: Highly hesitant
7–9: Deeply doubtful

Whatever your score… I'll be honest: these are all myths and misconceptions, and in some cases just flat out not true. I'm not here to convince you, or force you to do anything. But the idea that these myths might stop you from benefiting from the truly life-changing effects and benefits of meditation breaks my heart a little bit. Heck, maybe one of these myths almost stopped you picking up this book in the first place. Maybe it was even bought for you by someone who suspects you need it, but you're not yet quite sure.

But, as the meditation teacher and author Sharon Salzberg says, "We don't meditate to get better at meditating, we meditate to get better at life."[1]

And let me be clear: I'm not asking you to meditate because I think there's anything wrong with you now. As the meditation teacher Liza Kindred told me: "You are complete, you're just not finished."[2] I also don't want you to think the goal is to become a floating cloud of bliss, devoid of any negative emotion, unable to enjoy a cocktail because you're so "enlightened", earnest and boring.

I want you to learn to meditate *in a way that works for you*, because of the peace, insight and happiness that I trust it can bring to your life and to others around you. And in order to get those benefits, you have to actually *do it*. The meditation, I mean. I know – annoying, isn't it?

You can read this book and talk about meditation and listen to all the podcasts and highlight all the self-help books and download every single app and buy all the beautiful paper journals. But, unless you get over yourself and literally *sit through* the distractions, discomfort, resistance and ideas you have about the actual meditation, you aren't going to get very far. It's the sitting, and the failing, and the trying again that builds the muscle in the brain, which reroutes the pathways that builds up the cortexes that make the changes that help you stop being such a bitch to yourself. Learn to be on your own side and enjoy life.

If you want to experience the real benefits of meditation, you have to *meditate*. The good news is that science shows us that incredible benefits can be attained with just 10–30 minutes per day, in a matter of weeks. And, *even better news*, if you practise regularly, you can actually start to *enjoy* your practice and look forward to it. Trust me.

But I understand why people have these misconceptions. With something like meditation, it's easy to get the wrong idea.

But, as with most stereotypes, these ideas often tend not to be true – or, at least, they're only one narrow version of the whole story. So, let's investigate.

I'm not the kind of person who meditates

Hands up if you've ever thought this. I have, and I'm a meditation teacher! But there is not only one kind of person who meditates. As long as you're respectful and learn the practice with a genuine intention, and know that there's a lot you don't know, then there's no such thing as being – or not being – "the right kind of person". Pretty much anyone can meditate (and get the benefits from it) if they are willing to take the time to learn how.

I'd love to meditate, but I never have enough time

Welcome to one of the most annoying proverbs *ever*: "You should sit in meditation for 20 minutes a day, unless you're too busy, then you should sit for an hour."

But truly, the person who thinks they don't have enough time to meditate is, usually, the person who stands to benefit *most* from it. If that's you, then you're *human*. But I would argue that everyone has two minutes a day to notice their breath. Even if it's when you're on the toilet. *If you have time to scroll on your smartphone, you have time to learn to meditate.*

Let me ask you: Do you want to carve out time for your mental health, or not? I'm not trying to shame anyone. Time is precious. But if you suspect meditation might be really good for you, you can definitely find time to prioritize it. I always encourage my clients to see meditation as "time out" from their busy schedule and to-do list, rather than just another thing to add to it.

And if you *don't* take care of your mental health, then it's almost inevitable that it *will* catch up with you. Usually, for me, it's physical. I get migraines if I ignore my body's warning signs that it's burning out. Your signs might be different, but they do exist. If you think you don't have time to meditate for a few minutes a day, then what you're really saying is that you are not choosing to prioritize it right now. And that's OK – but it's not because you don't have time. (I know – tough love, so early on!)

I am mindful in other ways, so I don't need to meditate

Unpopular opinion, but "being mindful" isn't the same as actual meditation. The science shows that an actual formal meditation practice (i.e., sitting and doing the thing) is what makes the difference, physically, in our brains.

Being mindful is great. It helps. One of my clients recently said that she felt she had become "30% more mindful in all areas of her life". And that's bloody excellent. Doing things mindfully – paying attention, on purpose, without judgement, is great. It can bring you back to the present, which is super-powerful in itself. It's like refreshing a G&T with more tonic water. A nice top-up, but not the real thing. "Formal" meditation (as in, doing a focused practice) is the only thing that has been proven to actually make the difference, and make the actual physical changes we want to see in the brain. Mindfully painting or swimming is not exactly the same thing. I know, it sucks. But sadly, we can't get the six-pack without doing the sit-ups.

I've tried it and I was terrible at it, so I gave up

When a toddler tries to walk and falls over, it doesn't think, "Maybe this whole walking thing isn't for me. I'll stop trying." It gets up, and it tries again. This is the same. No-one is good at meditation when they start. Literally no-one. There's a reason I started this chapter with that Pema Chödrön quote. And *she's* a *Buddhist nun.*

Luckily though, the goal is not to empty our mind, think of nothing, and be totally calm. Being terrible at meditation is the *point*. Stop trying to be perfect and see what happens. Approach the absolute batshit stuff your brain throws at you with as much humour as you can.

When someone tells me they tried to meditate and their mind was so busy that "they couldn't do it", I want to give them a giant hug. *Because they're actually doing it right.* Meditation is the only thing I know of that you can actively fail at and know you're succeeding in the process. In fact, the point at which you notice your distraction is where the magic happens. Keep going. Slowly, you'll get a bit better. Your mind will stay attentive for two milliseconds, and then three. Then four. That's the practice. That's proof it's working.

Having a wellness routine is boring – I want to be spontaneous and free

Same. But you can be spontaneous, creative, interesting, routine-hating, go with the flow, enjoy life, drink alcohol, eat meat, swear, enjoy yourself, avoid every day being the same... and also meditate.

Despite associations with "focus", routine and vegan, teetotal retreats, meditation and who you are *now* are not mutually exclusive. Many people find that, even though they hate routine, the stillness and stress-relief that meditation can bring actually helps them stay sane without feeling constricted or bored.

Think about who you are now, and how that can fit in with meditation. See it as a part of who you already are. What parts of yourself do you already like or feel good about, which you can include or make good use of in your meditation and mindset routine?

- Are you curious?
- Do you enjoy getting organized and finding space?
- Are you actually quite introverted and enjoy your own company?
- Are you curious about psychology and how the mind works?

If you start to see your new "meditator" identity as part of the new habits you're trying to make, and part of who you already are anyway, it'll be way easier to make them stick.

Meditation has been whitewashed

Yes, it has. I don't agree with whitewashing anything, even though some people would see *me* as part of the problem. But I also believe just because some people have whitewashed meditation beyond recognition, that doesn't mean it cannot be learned or practised respectfully. See Chapter 15 for how.

Meditation makes you selfish and self-obsessed

I can see where this comes from. After all, meditation asks you to close your eyes and focus on yourself. Indeed, many people use meditation as a means to focus more on themselves, to figure out their own issues, and to untangle their inner struggles.

Firstly, this is no bad thing. Being more in touch with yourself after a lifetime of ignoring problematic emotions, distracting yourself with food, work, drinks, and being busy all the time, can be of huge benefit. But meditation shows us that the more we sit and understand the way we are, the more we understand the exact same in others, too.

Meditation might start with us becoming more self-obsessed, but if done correctly and consistently, it will actually lead to us becoming much less so. For all its marketing as a solo activity, meditation has actually long been practised in groups. Buddhists call their meditation community a "sangha," which loosely translates as an "association", "assembly" or "company". Meditation also allows you to join the great, global community of meditators. You may seem to be focusing on yourself, but you're actually part of a wider whole.

I don't need meditation: I'm pretty chill already

Are you lost in the wrong book? Tell me your secrets! And meditation isn't just about being chill. It has a host of benefits that go far beyond that.

I can't "live in the present"– I have stuff to do!

You can plan for the future or learn from the past and still live in the present as much as possible. For example, you have a flight to catch:

- Planning = packing your bag and leaving for the airport in good time.

- Worrying = hurriedly packing for every single possible season, taking too much in your suitcase, and spending hours stressing about all the things that could go wrong on the way to the airport.

If we choose the second option, we might completely ruin our day in the process, and arrive at the airport as a total wreck. Worrying may make us *feel* as though we are preparing. But this is just us trying to control the uncontrollable. See Chapter 5 for way more on this!

I'm afraid of what I'll find in my brain if I sit still and listen to my thoughts

I totally get you. Often we suspect there's an issue hovering in our mind, and we just think that if we don't give it the time of day, it might leave us alone. Even now, I am sometimes surprised by the absolute shite that my brain throws at me when I sit still for a few moments.

It can be song lyrics, memories of horrible moments in the playground when I was nine, or a patronizing conversation I had eight years ago with a colleague I haven't seen since. But, as hard as it sounds, sometimes the things we encounter during meditation are useful. They can be signs of things that are unresolved, and a signal that we need to be kind to ourselves or deal with an issue.

Of course, some people suffering from trauma, PTSD or serious mental illness may find meditation is not appropriate for them right now, at least not without a trained, trauma-sensitive teacher or psychiatrist. For them, what they find when they close their eyes may be genuinely scarring and re-traumatizing.

But for most of us, our brain simply taunts us with negative or bizarre or totally random thoughts, and that's normal.

But the best part? During your meditation sessions, *it doesn't matter*. You are learning to feel safe, no matter what your brain throws at you. The whole point is to see meditation as your *time away from* judging yourself. The real goal is not to *control* your thoughts, but to notice them, and let them float away again, coming back to the breath or body.

This gets easier. I am not advising that you "shut up and get on with it," or totally dismiss any worries or scary thoughts that you may have about sitting with yourself. But if your resistance feels more like, "I'm stressed, I don't want to, it's too uncomfortable, I can't!" then I would gently say, *you can*. You're safe, and you can always stop and take a break if you need to.

The more you practise, the better you will get at approaching the weird shit your brain contains, with compassion and curiosity. This, in turn, is likely to allow you to turn down the dial on it, too. It's a virtuous cycle.

3

A How-to Guide to Beginners' Meditation

(or, Put your Mind to It)

"Every action you take is a vote for the type of person you wish to become. No single instance will transform your beliefs, but as the votes build up, so does the evidence of your new identity."

James Clear, author

If you've read this far, I'm guessing you're at least ready to *try* to meditate. Maybe you've tried before. Maybe you're a few sessions in on your new meditation app and finding it tough. Maybe you're ready to go! Or perhaps you're still sceptical.

Finding the time, space, motivation and quiet can feel impossible, even when you want to. People often say to me, "I want to meditate, but my mind is too busy." But that's a bit like saying you're "too tired to sleep" or to "too hungry to eat".

That's why we do it. I know, because I first learned to meditate on the London Underground... at rush hour.

RUSH HOUR MEDITATION

I tell this story to anyone who worries they don't have the time, space or patience to meditate. If I can do it on an underground train, I promise you can do it where *you* are, too. For those first few years, I'd squeeze myself inside the train – packed in with a thousand other people – breathe in to avoid the closing doors, find something to balance against, ignore everyone and, in the few millimetres of space I had to move my thumb, press "play" on my meditation app.

Every day, I'd let the disgruntled commuters ebb and flow around me, as I closed my eyes for those few precious minutes. It wasn't easy. The train would stop regularly. I'd have to shuffle out of the way, and even open my eyes every few minutes to check I wasn't accidentally leaning on a door (or a person, eek!). But it worked. Minute by minute. For one particular visualization meditation, I figured out that if I pressed play at the start of my journey, I'd visualize reaching the top of a sunlit hiking trail in my mind at the exact same time as I'd reach the top of a real-life escalator. It felt brilliant.

Even though I'd changed nothing externally, meditation helped me feel confident and powerful, and able to visualize a happier life for myself – and no-one around me had any idea what was going on. I felt free. I'd emerge, blinking, from the dark of Victoria Underground Station, and feel ever-so-slightly more peaceful and ready for the day that lay before me. It wasn't magic, but it made my commute more bearable.

No matter how stressed I felt, how busy the train, or how many times I'd almost nod off, I'd try again and again – and slowly, slowly, I got better at it. I felt better. It became a habit. I'd almost look forward to getting on the Tube, just so I could put those headphones in, and breathe. In fact, my meditation became *so* associated with my commute that at the weekends, I struggled to find the discipline to do it.

That's how I realized that making new habits isn't about willpower, or how much you want it, or finding the exact right time or moment. It's about repetition, and not waiting until everything is perfect to start. If I had waited until I felt calm enough, ready enough, or had the perfect place or the perfect time to begin learning to meditate, I would never have got started.

Sure, by all means, buy a meditation cushion and candle, or go on a retreat. But if you're anything like me, you need to keep things simple. Tune out the BS and the excuses, and tune in to what you need. As the Arthur Ashe quote goes: "To achieve greatness, start where you are, use what you have, do what you can."

My flat in London at the time wasn't even big enough for me to have a full-size bed, let alone a dedicated meditation space. I didn't have a proper meditation cushion or mat, or the money to go on a retreat or to a fancy studio. I was so burned out that if I had sat down to meditate at home, I would have nodded off within seconds. What I needed was to cut the excuses. I needed to beat the overthinking, and my lack of willpower, and the self-flagellation, and just do it. That's the power of making things a habit, rather than relying on willpower. It takes all that noise and the emotional ups and downs out of the picture, and allows you to get the thing done.

This next section is all about helping you to do just that.

Meditation is not always easy – but it IS simple

The basic instruction is this:

Sit comfortably, notice your breath. If you get distracted, notice it, forgive yourself, and come back to it. Repeat. End.

To break it down even more:

1. Sit comfortably, but as upright and alert as you can.
2. Close your eyes or keep them slightly open.
3. Take a few deep breaths, and then breathe normally.
4. Notice where you can feel your breath physically (e.g., nose, chest, stomach, back)....
5. ... Bring your attention there, without judgement.
6. When your mind gets distracted, as soon as you realize, bring your focus back, *without judgement*.
7. Repeat 17 billion times until your session/patience ends.
8. Try again tomorrow. Repeat.

I recommend that for each suggested meditation in this book, you start with these steps, unless stated otherwise. But what if you struggle? Read on.

I'm so distracted, I can't do it!

Congratulations, you're doing it right! If you expect to stay focused or blissfully relaxed every time you sit down to meditate, then it's bad news, my friend. Our minds will never, ever be blank or empty. "Emptying your mind" is not the goal. The goal is to focus our attention on something specific, for a certain amount of time, and *when* (not *if*) we get distracted, bring it back.

But getting distracted *can* be annoying. So I also recommend:

- Slowing down: get weirdly curious. Pretend you've got a tiny magnifying glass and zoom into the physical feelings of your breath and body even more.
- Noticing every tiny movement of that inhale, that exhale.
- Tuning into the sensations of your fingertips as if you were trying to discern individual grains of sand.
- Filling your attention *so* much that you don't have any extra mental bandwidth to get distracted or bored. Try again. Repeat.

What if I still struggle?

The only way out is through. You'll get better at it, I promise. Of course, this doesn't mean that you should ignore your moods, or push through genuine pain to force yourself to do something you really don't want to/can't do. This isn't about ignoring your body and mind.

You're not supposed to be actively suffering through meditation. Any intense pain, flashbacks, sweating, out-of-body-experiences, or anything that feels truly negative, can be a sign of trauma, and is known as "dysregulation". It should absolutely not be ignored. If this happens, stop, seek medical help and/ or get the face-to-face advice of an expert who is specifically trained in healing trauma.

But if you find that you're feeling something like, "Wow, this is harder than I'd like, I would rather be, well, doing *anything* except being with myself right now." then you're doing it right. Be gentle, and try again.

This is hard. I thought meditation was supposed to be *relaxing*?

I cannot stress this enough: meditation is not always about relaxing. If you want a bubble bath or a nap, by all means have one. But *this* is a lifelong mental health practice. Even 12-plus years into it, I still have terrible days. I fell asleep to a guided track only last week, and only realized because the teacher's voice told me my time was up. Some days, it's great. I feel aware, at peace, present, purposeful, focused and calm. But, mainly, I'm distracted. I zone out. I get a song lyric stuck in my head on a loop, or I write a mental to-do list. Focus. Breathe. Repeat. That's the process.

Once again, *noticing that you're distracted means it's working*. The important thing is not to let this feeling that it's hard derail your progress. One of my favourite cartoons is of a Buddhist monk meditating, saying, "Come on, Inner Peace, I don't have all day." But, sadly, you can't order inner peace on Amazon Prime.

For many of us, meditation feels like a pain in the butt, and something that we struggle through, rather than enjoy, especially at first. You're doing it right. Keep going.

Why meditate if it's hard? Life is hard enough

I hear you. Life is short. Why do something that you don't enjoy? Indeed, many of us come to meditation because we're suffering from stress, anxiety, overthinking, self-doubt, depression, fear or mild trauma, and we're looking for relief.

So why do this, if it's just *another* difficult thing? Dan Harris, founder of the meditation brand 10% Happier, often says meditation can easily lapse into an "eating your vegetables" attitude.[1] It can feel like the boiled broccoli on the plate of life. We know we *should* eat it – but why, when ice cream exists? But as the meditation teacher Cory Muscara wrote, "Meditation isn't about feeling good. It's about paying attention with good awareness. Plot twist: that will eventually feel good."[2] He's not wrong.

So doing this hard thing will make me feel better?

Yes. In fact, cognitive behavioural therapy (CBT) uses what's called a "thoughts, feelings, behaviour" cycle to explain this. It shows that shifting our thoughts and feelings can positively impact on our behaviour, and therefore our mood, and that we need a combination of enjoyment and achievement to feel our best. Working at our desk for an hour *and* taking a walk. Scheduling in a tough workout *and* a night on the sofa. Such contrasts can shift up negative or circular thought patterns in our mind and help us feel better overall.

As always, balance is key. We're all a mixture of "carrot" and "stick". As my old gym used to have written on the wall: "'I regretted that workout,' said no-one, ever." It's cheesy, but it's true. Getting started is the hardest part. Staying consistent and carrying when it doesn't feel good, and when nothing seems to be working, is the second hardest part. One of the most powerful lessons I ever learned when training in CBT is the idea that we don't have to *feel* like doing something to do it. Often, the motivation comes *after* we begin, not the other way around.

And the key is consistency. The tiny gains and improvements, day in, day out, make the difference. It's all about endurance, the showing up when you don't feel like it. Just as the writer Glennon Doyle, (and one of my favourite podcasters, Nicole Antoinette of Real Talk Radio[3]), says, "We can do hard things."[4] Not because "life is pain", or "no pain, no gain" or any of that self-flagellating bullshit. But because sticking at something that's difficult can actually help us feel good, and build trust in ourselves. Building up the habit of meditation can boost our self-worth and our relationship with ourselves, day after day.

Some days, meditation might be the only thing you do that feels productive. Some days, when my anxiety is high, I think, "Well, if I only do ten minutes of meditation today, at least I'll have done *something*". Showing up is not just about meditating. It's about not breaking a promise we made to ourselves. Establishing these "habit loops" – completing something we said we would – gives our brain little hits of dopamine, which helps us feel happier, and more motivated to keep going. It's a virtuous cycle, which helps you to stay consistent in other areas of your life too. If you prove to yourself you can stick to this then you can, in theory, stick to anything.

THE WINE GLASS ANALOGY

Beware the temptation to try too hard during meditation. I know, I know, we're ambitious people who like to do stuff properly. But when we start a new habit, it can be so tempting to place an overwhelming expectation on ourselves to be "the best" at it. And before long, we're sitting there, meditating for dear life, willing inner peace to make itself known, and getting nothing in return but a big old tension headache. That's the quickest way to make meditation feel stressful, like something *else* on your to-do list, rather than something that can act as a nice break from it.

The solution is to try less hard. Imagine you're holding a crisp glass of whatever you fancy. If you hold it too tightly, the glass could break. Too loosely, and it will fall out your hand. We're aiming for just enough grip to hold the glass... but not so much that we won't be invited back.

Admittedly, when you're a beginner, it's better to be *too* focused than not focused enough. But I prefer to think of it as curiosity, rather than intense focus. Think of your attention like an interested and twinkly professor – more '90s Robin Williams than '80s Jack Nicholson.

Getting started

When should I meditate, and what do I need?

At its simplest, you only need your breath, body and mind. Nothing else. No fancy cushions, studios, bells, bowls, gongs, crystals, candles, noise-cancelling headphones, expensive gadgets or phone apps. That stuff is nice, but it's not *necessary*.

Everywhere you look, there will be someone telling you that their way is the best – that you must meditate at 5am and sit *just so*. But there's no set rule. The perfect time and way to meditate is when and how you will *actually do it*.

But, of course, there are some things you can do to make your new habit more consistent.

Making meditation a habit: My top tips

- Decide when you're going to do it, and commit to the same time each day. Morning commute, lunchtime, before dinner. Whenever works for you.
- Attach your new habit to something else you always do. That might be while brushing your teeth, or after your shower. This acts as a cue and makes it easier to form a habit.
- Sit/stand wherever feels comfortable. You do not have to twist your legs into the lotus position unless you want to. Stay upright and alert, but feel comfortable. I could never meditate lying down as I'd be asleep in seconds, but the brilliant meditation teacher and author Sebene Selassie recommends it[5] – so find whatever feels best for you.
- Find somewhere relatively quiet, if you can. But even if you can't, that's OK. You can actually make noise part of your meditation. As I discovered last week, there's nothing quite like meditating next to a window when someone outside is using a chainsaw on a tree. Sigh.
- Start small, and work up. Start with five good breaths, or set a timer for one minute, and try that. Then add

five minutes. Repeat until 10-20 minutes feels more manageable (trust me, it will). It's better to do ten minutes a day than an hour, once.

- Work with yourself. If you're not a morning person, then don't expect yourself to suddenly be able to meditate before dawn. Equally, if you know that you tend to feel sleepy after 4pm, try to meditate before then. Again – whatever works for you.

Tracking your progress

I've put this in a new section because it can be genius if you're getting started (and it can help you get back on track even if you're a long-time meditator).

Tracking your sessions builds consistency and a pattern, and encourages you to keep going. All it means is that whenever you successfully complete a session, you make a note of it, or tick it off on a calendar, and build up a record, or visual proof of your habit.

I recommend keeping it simple. Try the following:

- Apps, such as Headspace[6] and 10% Happier[7], which keep track for you.
- Habit-tracking apps, such as Momentum[8] or Productive.[9]
- Set an appointment for meditating on your calendar every day and tick it off when it's done.
- Pen and paper also works! This is my favourite method. Print off a paper calendar, and stick it on the fridge. When you do a session, tick it off with a bright highlighter.

Before long, it enforces your habit; you don't want to break that promise to yourself or break that streak. It feels good to build up a consistent, visual pattern; it gives you structure, and proves something to yourself: "Look at me, showing up for myself. Maybe I *actually am* worth something! Maybe I *can* do new and hard things!" Scientists have called this "closing the habit loop". Setting the goal opens the loop, doing the habit continues it, and ticking off the session provides confirmation that the habit has been done, thereby closing the loop.

Taking quick notes (e.g., "Felt drowsy today," or "Really inspired today,") or scoring your session out of ten, also allows you to see deeper patterns. For example, if you notice you miss your session every Sunday, or fall asleep every Tuesday, you can think about why that might be, and tweak your schedule accordingly. Making notes or scoring your sessions isn't about striving for a perfect score or trying to be perfect. It's just about noticing that the quality of your sessions will fluctuate. You might have one great day, then a terrible one. It's normal. Tracking helps you see this over time, and not get discouraged.

Reward yourself

When starting something new, it can feel daunting. Forever is a long time, especially when viewed from the start of a new habit. So instead, begin with a timeframe that feels manageable.

- For example, set yourself a goal of meditating for ten minutes, for five days straight. Or seven. Or 21, 30, 60, 90. Work up.
- Track it. And *then*? Give yourself a reward when you stick to it.

Depending on your motivation style, you may frame it as getting a treat if you succeed, or not getting one if you don't. Most of us like a mixture of both. Do whatever you need to get it done, without being too harsh on yourself!

To help, I always advise my clients to take The 5 Love Languages Quiz, which was first developed by counsellor Dr Gary Chapman.[10] You can take it on his website.[11] The quiz was first designed to help couples show love toward each other in a way each person truly understands, but it works for ourselves, too.

According to Dr Chapman, there are five types of love languages:

1. Words of affirmation
2. Gifts
3. Acts of service
4. Quality time
5. Physical touch

Once you know your main types, I recommend choosing one or two rewards for yourself from each, and picking one in advance for when you reach your goal. Knowing your types is key, as there's no point making your reward a bubble bath because you *think* that's what self-care looks like when, actually, you would much prefer a massage, a glass of wine, dinner out or a night in alone with a good book.

Knowing your love language means you'll be more likely to pick a reward that works for you. Here are some of my favourite ideas, organized by love language type:

Words of affirmation

- Buy a new notebook to write powerful affirmations in, such as "I stick to my goals", "I am a badass", "I can do hard things".
- Call/meet your most supportive friend for a celebratory chat.
- Tell your partner that you'd appreciate their outspoken support or words of encouragement.
- Stick fancy Post-It notes with affirmations written on them, around the house.
- One of my clients even designs simple postcards with encouraging phrases on them, on the free design website Canva, and sends them to herself every week!

Gifts

- Treat yourself to a fancy scented candle.
- Purchase an item from your Amazon wish list.
- Pick up that book you've been meaning to read for ages.
- Sign up for a subscription to a new monthly gift box.

Acts of service

- Get a takeaway instead of cooking.
- Ask your partner to cook for you instead.
- Hire a one-off or regular cleaning service.
- Sort out a rota for taking the bins out/cleaning the bathroom.

Physical touch

- Book in for a massage. One of my clients said meditation felt "like getting a mind and brain massage," so she booked herself a full-body one for each month of meditation she completed.

- Use a luxurious moisturizer.
- Soak in a hot, velvety bubble bath and wrap yourself in a soft, warm towel afterwards.

Quality time
- Spend an evening with your partner, no phones allowed.
- Go for a long-overdue dinner with a friend.
- Snuggle up on the sofa for a night of watching/reading/crafting whatever you want.

Your reward doesn't have to be fancy or expensive. It just needs to be meaningful to you, to remind you how well you're doing.

Plan for missed days
You know what they say about the best laid plans. No matter how perfectly you schedule your sessions, and track them, life will get in the way sometimes.

For example, one of my clients used to do her meditation when she came home from work, before making dinner. It was perfect. But on the few nights when she went out to eat with friends or had an evening work event, she would miss her usual meditation slot. Another client woke up at 4am one day with her head full of ideas, and by her usual meditation time – 8am – she was already four hours and two coffees deep into the day, and had missed her meditation completely... which turned into a week of missed sessions.

But that's life. Perhaps your disruption is a lovely thing, such as a holiday. Or maybe it's less lovely – your child or your dog is sick. But the key is to plan for this unexpected disruption to your routine as much as you can. Think about:

- If you miss your morning session, when will you find ten minutes later in the day?
- Do you have a work event later so you won't get time to meditate? What about a one-off session during your lunch break?
- A friend asks you to dinner out of the blue, but you usually meditate in the evening, and there's no time for a backup plan? No worries. One missed day won't ruin your habit. Enjoy your night!

Get back on it the next day and keep on keeping on.

Setting new habits – whether it's meditation, jogging or even just drinking more water – is supposed to help *improve* your life, not make it harder. The more boring, difficult or new something is, the less sustainable. Expect to fail every now and again, so that when you do, you'll be able to say, "That's life!" and carry on.

Avoid "all or nothing" thinking

You know that moment when you think you've screwed something up, so you say "Fuck it!" and throw the whole thing away? Usually, it happens when we've made a mistake, or fallen off the wagon on a new habit. We think: "I've ruined it now, I'll never get this, no point continuing." We see the situation starkly, in black and white. It's a way of protecting ourselves, but in reality, it's textbook self-sabotage. We throw in the towel so that we don't have to do the difficult work of admitting that we screwed up, but still need to carry on. In that moment, it can feel easier to give up. But if we do, we'll delay getting the benefits we want.

Just as if we're trying to eat healthily, eating one chocolate chip cookie doesn't mean we should give up and eat deep-fried cheeseburgers for the rest of the day or week. One way to combat this is to use the phrase "and". For example: "I missed a session yesterday and I'm going to try again today." or, "I felt like that session was terrible and I know that it still counts." It's both, not either/or. Rewiring your mind is a lifelong practice. That's why it's so important to fit it into your lifestyle, and to give yourself a break when, inevitably, you fall off the wagon.

Practising meditation is as much about being kind to yourself when you "fail" as when you succeed. *You cannot hate yourself into change.* And "failing" at meditation *is* the practice. I cannot stress this enough. But as Samuel Beckett wrote: "Ever tried. Ever failed. No matter. Try again. Fail again. Fail better."[12]

I've got to be honest: when I first read that quote, I thought: "OK for you, Samuel Beckett, the rest of us need to succeed." Because if you're anything like me, this idea feels mind-blowing and a little *suspect*, because it turns everything I was brought up to believe about achievement on its head. For us perfectionists, who stop ourselves from even *trying* something new for fear of failure, the idea that failing can make us better, can feel backwards. But when we finally realize, it's a huge weight off our shoulders, and can help us be more daring in the rest of our life.

If we know that failure isn't the disaster we once feared it was, we might be less afraid of taking that first step.

Remember, the goal is not to be the world's best meditator. The goal is to keep trying, and to be kinder to yourself as you go. You're going to mess up. And that's how we improve. If you ever needed a safe space to practise that idea, then meditation is it.

GET UNSTUCK: FAQS

What if I keep falling asleep?

Totally normal. But *constantly* falling asleep is a sign of a few things, namely that you're sleep deprived. If you keep falling asleep whenever you sit still, this is a massive sign from your body that you need more – or better – sleep. Start there! (See Chapter 9).

What do I do with my arms?

Whatever feels comfortable. Some might hold their hands together in their lap, some keep the ends of their thumbs touching. Others might opt for a "mudra", which is where you hold the fingertips of two fingers together – think of the clichéd "meditation on a beach" pose. Personally, I like to hold my hands in my lap, as it feels natural, or I might let my palms face upwards, as a sort of physical metaphor for being "open". Whatever works for you.

I keep missing days, no matter what I do

Again, this is *totally normal*. Try and try again. I still sometimes miss days too, especially Saturdays if I sleep in, or can't be bothered. But if you can't get consistent for love nor money, and keep dropping off for days, weeks or months, then we've maybe got a deeper issue. Ask yourself:

- Why do you want to meditate in the first place?
- What pain – such as anxiety, worry, fear, overthinking, bad sleep, lack of confidence, etc. – are you hoping to improve by doing this?
- How would your life feel if you fixed that pain? What would you be able to *be, do or have* if you prioritized this?
- Can you give yourself a more incentivizing reward? Or buddy up with someone, perhaps?

Remember, you don't *have* to do this. It's a choice. So get honest with yourself.

I don't like focusing on my breath – it makes me hyperventilate or panic

This is quite common among new meditators. Deep breathing can stimulate our parasympathetic nervous system, reduce our blood pressure, and help us to feel calm. But, for some people, paying attention to their breath can cause panic, worry about whether they're breathing "right", or even prompt hyperventilation.

A major reason that guided meditations might ask us to focus on the breath is because it's always there, and it's portable. But you can use another "anchor" to focus on instead. This could be a part of your body, a particular texture on your clothing, or even certain sounds. Some like to use a small, handheld object, such as a soft toy or a smooth stone. You could, say, use your morning coffee cup, and use the texture, warmth and taste as your anchor.

One of my clients started to meditate in the shower every day, and used the sensation of the water on her skin as her "anchor". Whatever helps you train your attention and doesn't trigger you, works. Eventually, everyone may be able to use the breath, but if you can't do it at first, that's OK.

Is using guided tracks bad? Should I be aiming to meditate alone, unguided?

There is no right or wrong here. Using a guided meditation track doesn't necessarily make you a "newbie", or mean you're not meditating properly. Guided tracks can be useful when you're starting out, and help you in years to come. I often use them to stay focused on a particularly difficult day, or when learning from a new teacher or technique. Some people love to meditate completely alone, no guided tracks at all. Some use recordings of bells or a timer, but no speech. Some use nature sounds or music.

With all of this, the main thing – always – is to find what works for you.

PART TWO

MEDITATION IN PRACTICE

4

Meditation for
Self-Compassion

(or, How to Stop Being Such a Bitch to Yourself)

*"You've been criticising yourself for years and it
hasn't worked. Try approving of yourself and see what
happens."*

Louise L. Hay, author, and founder of publisher Hay House

Let's imagine for a second that you have a running coach.
Imagine you're sitting in your living room, when your running
coach shows up. He's jabbing a finger at you, telling you to "Get
your fat arse out there and run!"

That *might* shock and annoy you enough to get you off the
sofa. You'd probably be out that door with your running shoes on
pretty damn sharpish. But then imagine that your coach *stayed*
angry. Imagine that he kept telling you that you weren't working
hard enough. Eventually, you're going to feel worse and even
more unmotivated. You'll probably end up stopping completely,

telling the coach to fuck right off, or both. You may have got out of the door, but now you're going nowhere fast, you feel like shit, and you're not even any closer to being a better runner.

Now, imagine that your coach encouraged you instead. He told you how brilliant it is that you got outside, and reminded you of how incredibly great you're going to feel when you finish. Imagine if your coach admitted that, yes, the run might be tough, but that you're getting better, and that if you keep trying, even when it feels difficult, you'll absolutely succeed. How much more likely would you be to get back out there?

Unless you're a total masochist who loves being shouted at, I'm guessing the answer is, a *lot* more likely. Maybe you'd even look forward to running, rather than feeling like a failure the whole time. That's the power of rewiring your inner critic through meditation – even if, at the beginning, it's a bit of a pain in the arse. Because life feels so much easier when you don't have a rude "coach" criticizing you constantly in your head.

In fact, that's how I recommend approaching meditation itself: try, fail, try, fail, be kind and encouraging to yourself, speak to yourself with compassion, rest a bit, stretch, try again. That's the practice. And it can apply to pretty much your whole life. Breathe. Try again. Build a safe space inside your own body and mind, transform the way that you speak to yourself, and know that no matter what, you *are* good enough and resilient enough to stay standing. Breathe. Repeat.

If you take only *one* thing away from this book, let it be this: you are of value; you are worth existing, loving, taking up space, and being exactly whoever the fuck you are (without hurting others!), simply because you are alive, human and yourself.

You may have made some less-than-great decisions in the past. You may have elements of yourself that you're less-than-proud of, or things you'd like to change. But that doesn't alter the constant fact: you are good enough and worth loving, simply for being you. End.

That's it. That's the end of the chapter.

OK, obviously not. Because if it were that simple, we'd all have done it by now.

And imagine the industries that would fall if everyone walked around with a safe, certain, gentle and steadfast belief in their own value! There are entire sectors of society dedicated to making us feel that our lives aren't good enough, encouraging us to spend money on things we don't need! Because *not feeling enough* is built into our very society. It's so common as to almost appear as an unavoidable part of the human experience.

A 2019 study found that eight in ten millennials (aged 22–38) thought they were "not good enough", three-quarters felt "overwhelmed", and 79% said these feelings had impacted their mental health. The same poll found that the women asked were more likely to not feel good enough (82%) compared to the men (73%).[1] These are not small numbers.

As the meditation teacher (and one of *my* teachers, too) Adreanna Limbach, author of *Tea and Cake with Demons: A Buddhist Guide to Feeling Worthy*,[2] told me on my podcast:

> *"Something that I've noticed for years is that, regardless of where the women I coach are from, something that*

*comes up consistently is a feeling of not being 'enough'.
All different ages, all different beliefs, backgrounds and
socioeconomic status, and religions and philosophies. It
couldn't be any more diverse.*

*"They use lots of different language to describe this
feeling of not knowing enough or not feeling prepared
enough, or not feeling pretty enough, or not feeling like
they had enough resources or enough education, or this
overwhelming sense of 'not enoughness', both in their
exterior life, but also internalized. It was this question of,
'Who do I think I am?'*

*"And then I realized: 'I'm not the only one who feels
this way.' It's systemic. This is across the globe. It's so
universal."*[3]

That's why I wholeheartedly subscribe to the fantastic Caroline
Caldwell quote: "In a society that profits from your self-doubt,
liking yourself is a rebellious act."[4]

Accept you are "enough"

Buddhism and meditation tell us that we are enough. They call
this "basic goodness". Our goal with meditation and mindful
living is to remember to wake up to that goodness, and live as
full an expression of that as we can everyday, with compassion
for ourselves and others.

Self-compassion is basically the principle that your own
"enoughness" rests inside you, that it cannot and will not be

found externally, and that you are already enough, exactly as you are, with no need to prove or change a thing. As Dr Kristen Neff, a foremost researcher in the concept of *self*-compassion, who literally wrote the book on it, writes:

> *"Mindfulness brings us back to the present moment and provides... balanced awareness that forms the foundation of self-compassion. Like a clear pool without ripples, mindfulness perfectly mirrors what's occurring, without distortion. Rather than becoming lost in our own personal soap opera, mindfulness allows us to view our situation with greater perspective and helps to ensure that we don't suffer unnecessarily."*[5]

I happen to believe that *this* is the holy grail of meditation and even life itself: enabling good, sensitive, self-doubting people to truly believe in their inherent, constant goodness. Everything comes back to that. I honestly believe that no matter the problem, the question, the trauma, the violence, the evil, the rage, the pain, the confusion, the uncertainty, the fear... the answer is compassion.

People without compassion or self-compassion are easy to spot. They usually treat others as badly as they treat themselves. As the expression goes: "Hurt people hurt people." Scratch the surface, and you'll usually find that someone who treats you badly is struggling just as much, if not more, themselves. When we hate ourselves, we behave like that. It doesn't feel good, and it's not conducive to a successful, fulfilled life.

That's why it's so important to tend to our inner voice and cultivate our own compassion. It makes everything feel easier, and we can move through the world more happily, treating others as we wish to be treated, and doing things with real love. We're no longer acting from a place of pain, but from a place of solid self-belief.

Unlearn bad habits

While that sounds nice, it doesn't necessarily make it any easier for us to *truly believe* that we are worthy. It can take years to unlearn decades of social conditioning and advertising. So many of us will tear our lives and relationships apart, and distract ourselves to death by doomscrolling through social media for hours, before we ever get still enough to examine why we're so afraid of being alone with the voices in our own heads, and why we never ever feel like anything we do, say, buy or achieve is good enough.

Your meditation session might be the *one time in the day* when you allow yourself to sit still enough to hear what those inner voices are saying, and reframe and rewire them to be kinder and more helpful. As the actor Anna Kendrick once famously tweeted: "Oh god. I just realized I'm stuck with me my whole life."[6] And if you're stuck with yourself your whole life – which, spoiler, you *are* – then isn't it a good idea to work on making yourself a nice person to hang out with?

A NOTE ON "SELF-LOVE"

A caveat: in the UK, the word "self-love" can prompt a chuckle, because it sounds more like a night in with a vibrator than a synonym of self-compassion. And yet, I use the word anyway, because it's the simplest way to explain what we're trying to do.

I used to think that it was just us stiff-upper-lip Brits who can't cope with terms such as "self-love". But Dan Harris of meditation brand 10% Happier, who is American, calls the term "ooey-gooey", and outwardly squirms at how saccharine it sounds, so it's not just us.

Personally, I try to use phrases like "giving yourself a break", "being on your own side", or "not being such a bitch to yourself", because those make most sense to me. So if you don't want to think of it as "self-love", then don't!

Love yourself, but for real this time

I must admit that I get frustrated with all the self-help books and magazine articles that tell us "all" we need to do is "love ourselves", and our problems will be solved. While we like the Instagram quotes that say, "You Are Enough", and it feels *nice* for a bit, pretty soon we're back to square one, with that familiar itch of not feeling good enough.

It turns out, there's a ginormous gap between *knowing* you need to love yourself, and actually *doing it*. Learning how to love yourself goes way deeper, and gets way darker, than chanting affirmations in the mirror, liking a photo, and telling yourself you'll never have a negative thought, ever again.

Thankfully, despite learning to love yourself being one of *the toughest things* to do, I am happy to report that mindfulness and meditation are the only things I've ever discovered that give us practical ways to actually make that shift. Tangibly, the repeated act of daily meditation, and the physical rewiring of the brain that it causes, helps us to unlearn the years – decades, even – of internal mental patterns and capitalistic conditioning that tell us that we're not enough. Practices such as "loving-kindness" meditation (or "metta") massively help build improved self-compassion. It's basically the Buddhist version of "You can't fill from an empty cup."

Yet, I believe that the importance of self-compassion often gets lost among some meditation teachers' obsession with "awareness" and being in the present. Self-compassion isn't an extra bonus to being self-aware – it is the whole practice. Because while the definition of mindfulness, as defined by Jon Kabat-Zinn, may be "paying attention, in the present moment, on purpose, without judgement",[7] meditation goes much further than that. Without compassion, awareness just leads to, er, more awareness, and not much else. That's better than nothing, but what's the point of noticing how mean the voice in our head is being to us without learning to change it?

Mindfulness without self-compassion is like a car without a key. It's ready to go, it's full of potential, and it might give you shelter, but it's getting you nowhere fast. In fact, when many people start meditating, they often say that their stress and anxiety gets *worse* rather than better, because they're now so *aware* of how stressed and mean to themselves they are, and it feels rubbish. Without self-compassion, we're stuck feeling like crap, without knowing what to do about it.

In fact, when we talk about "awareness" and "acceptance" in meditation, we definitely don't mean "resignation" or giving up. As author, poet, activist and educator Sonya Renee Taylor explains in her book, *The Body Is Not An Apology: The Power of Radical Self-Love*, we are actually aiming to go beyond the usual "shrug shoulders-OK-but-not-great", resigned meaning of the word "acceptance".

She writes:

> "[I am] not going to help you with self-acceptance. Not because self-acceptance isn't useful, but because I believe there is a port far beyond the island of self-acceptance, and I want us to go there. Think back to all the times you accepted something and found it completely uninspiring."[8]

Becoming more aware and "noticing what is and letting it go", doesn't mean becoming acutely aware of our stresses and struggles, and giving up any hope of changing them. For some, finding awareness is already major. We're literally rewiring the brain, remember. It takes a while.

But, once we've stopped hating ourselves, compassion allows us to not only *notice* critical thoughts, but question and reframe them into something kinder, and more useful. Using tools such as mindfulness and loving-kindness, we can practise being less of a bitch to ourselves, and be much more caring, open, forgiving and loving.

As my Buddhism teacher Lodro Rinzler writes in his book, *The Buddha Walks Into a Bar*: "No teacher said the best way to create inner change is to be a prick to yourself."[9]

Despite all this, I know that when you tell people they need to love themselves, there are some common questions that come up.

If I love myself as I am, won't I lose all my motivation?

Often, people imagine that if they ever love themselves for who they are, then they'll lose any need to change or improve, and they'll lie in bed all day, without motivation. Firstly, I would argue: *What's wrong with that, sometimes?* I can recommend lying in bed feeling good about yourself. It's a lot nicer than lying in bed stressing about everything you haven't done and everything you hate about yourself.

But I get it. We're ambitious. We have big goals. It's a perfectly legit concern to think that if we work on feeling good enough as we are, we risk taking away any impetus to achieve anything else. The fatal flaw with this belief is that it's based on the idea that your ambition comes entirely from the sense that you're not good enough and you haven't achieved enough yet. But just like the example of the runner at the beginning of this chapter, being driven by that sense of lacking might get you off the sofa initially, but it won't feel good, and it *certainly* won't keep you going when things get tough.

Your negative inner voice and anxiety aren't what push you to get shit done. *You* do that. The negative inner voice and anxiety is just making it harder. Recent scientific research by neuroscientist Dr Judson Brewer, whose research on the brain spans 20 years, even *proves* this. As he explains in his recent book, *Unwinding Anxiety*:

"Our brains have tricked us into thinking that we need to be anxious to get things done and perform well. Anxiety doesn't actually improve performance. The key component in the process of unwinding anxiety is learning to be curious."[10]

If you stop motivating yourself with self-hatred and a fear of not being good enough, and start pushing yourself from a place of peace – cheer yourself on minus the constant inner criticism – you'll find your creativity and drive will *flourish*, not fail. If we practise sitting with ourselves, we learn to tell the difference between striving for something we want and striving for something because other people think we should want it. One feels good, the other feels like pushing water up a cliff. Luckily, you can accept and like who you are, and realize that there are still things you want to improve on and achieve.

And if you *do* find that your entire motivation for doing something is based purely on a sense of not feeling good enough, and having to prove to yourself and to others that you're just as good or better than they are, then I'd gently suggest that you may need to get some new goals, and really ask yourself what you want, and why. When you feel good enough about yourself, it's so much easier to pick goals that are aligned with your values, that make you feel good at your core, and that you can work on with much more ease and flow.

But what if I've experienced trauma – can I still love myself then?

The short answer is "yes", but it may need a little more time, and sensitivity.

I am not a trained trauma specialist, so if you want or need to dig deeper on this then I highly recommend the work of trauma-sensitive mindfulness teacher and writer, David A. Treleaven, and seeking out the support of a fully-trained trauma specialist. Through David's amazing work, I have learned that trauma can affect how effectively meditation helps us to cultivate self-compassion, and is at the root of why so many of us find it so difficult to love ourselves.

Firstly, let me define what I mean by "trauma". I spoke to Jessi Beyer, motivational speaker, trauma survivor and author of *How To Heal: A Practical Guide To Nine Natural Therapies You Can Use To Release Your Trauma*,[11] about how to know if trauma is affecting you. She told me:

"I define trauma as a very emotionally raw event that sticks with you into future days in your life. For some people, having a car accident is really traumatic and they

will never get behind the wheel again. Other people, they
drive again the next day.
    "The key thing is that is that it's way more emotion than
normal. Everything is wrong. You're on high alert. You can't
just conclude the event and then go about your life. It stays
with you in cinematic form. It holds on in your body."[12]

Jessi also explains how trauma is not only the big things that
happen to you – what she calls "big T" trauma. Trauma can also
build up over time, like a thousand papercuts that one day sever
your arm. She calls this "little t" trauma. She says:

"'Big T' traumas are the things that everyone thinks about
as traumatic: domestic abuse, a car accident, being sexually
assaulted, having a child die. Everyone recognizes those as
really difficult. But 'little t' traumas are things like your mum or
dad making a negative remark about you repeatedly in your
childhood, or losing a pet. It can add up. And depending on
the person, a 'little t' trauma can feel like a 'big T' trauma."[13]

Trauma specialist and psychotherapist Pat Ogden has written,
"Any experience that is stressful enough to leave us feeling
helpless, frightened, overwhelmed, or profoundly unsafe is
considered a trauma."[14]
    By these definitions, I believe that many of us are carrying
around some form of trauma in our everyday lives, maybe without
even knowing. We don't think to call what we've suffered "trauma"
because we don't think our lives are "bad enough", but then we
wonder why we constantly self-sabotage, or find it so difficult

to believe that we're good enough. As the author and therapist Lori Gottlieb says so insightfully, "There's no hierarchy of pain. Suffering shouldn't be ranked, because pain is not a contest."[15]

In some cases, self-sabotage and "talking ourselves down" are coping mechanisms that we have discovered to keep ourselves safe. As a 2018 study into trauma-informed mental health services puts it, "The fundamental shift in providing support using a trauma-informed approach is to move from thinking, 'What is wrong with you?' to considering 'What happened to you?'"[16] Much of the time, our negative thoughts and lack of self-worth can be traced to a particular incident in the past, usually (but not always) in childhood. Some therapists, meditation teachers and hypnosis specialists call this "inner child work". It's the idea that we can link problems with our self-worth now to things that happened – or didn't happen – when we were kids. This doesn't always solve everything, but it can offer insight.

We may have been bullied at school, so we now avoid others, even when we crave connection. Or we might have grown up in a loud and argumentative household, so we avoid confrontation as an adult, even when there are things that really need to be said. Glory-Anne Jones, a life coach and hypnotherapist, told me:

"When we meet our inner child, who has been hurt emotionally, maybe they feel worthless, like they have no place in this world, or should never speak up.

"Maybe we didn't get the love we needed when we were a child... but as the adult now, you can embrace that inner child. You're learning to love yourself. Many people

look for love outside of themselves. But if they don't know how to love themselves first, then it might be there, but they might miss it, or it's not ever going to fit, because they didn't turn that dial on themselves that says, 'Hi, I love myself, who else is ready to love with me?'

"If you're able to go deeper, through meditation and hypnosis, you're able to see more, because you don't have that interruption from that conscious mind that is saying, 'You don't deserve this healing. You don't deserve this love.'

"But our conscious mind needs to understand, 'I do deserve this love. And I do deserve a new start. I am an amazing being. I'm not here to be in this pit of despair and hurt.'"

At its most raw and powerful, meditation can help us love ourselves *even in the presence of trauma*, especially if it's with a "small t". And even "big T" trauma can be helped through meditation, with the help of a skilled teacher.

As David A. Treleaven writes in his book, *Trauma-Sensitive Mindfulness*: "Basic mindfulness practice is safer and more effective when it's paired with an understanding of trauma."[17]

Meditation for self-compassion can give you permission to stop, breathe, feel safe within your mind and body, and finally allow yourself to go to those places that you usually keep hidden, approaching them with tenderness, forgiveness and love, not fear.

Figuring out *why* we struggle with self-compassion isn't just another way to feel bad about ourselves. It's an invitation to identify where we might have developed unhealthy or unhelpful coping mechanisms, and why we struggle to believe we're good enough. So we can finally learn to forgive ourselves for that, and take a healthier and happier path as a result.

Isn't saying "I'm good enough no matter what" just letting yourself off the hook, or promoting false positivity?

Self-compassion – and even meditation itself – is not about simply ignoring your feelings, pretending everything is OK, or covering them up with empty or saccharine phrases. Meditation can be soothing and calming, yes, but it can also *start to repair what's causing the negative feelings in the first place*. It's both symptomatic relief and cure. It's not about feeling relaxed all the time, ignoring all your troubles, or pretending you'll never have another negative thought again. Using practices such as meditation in this way is known as "spiritual bypassing", or "toxic positivity", and both are dangerous for our own mental health, and for society at large.

TOXIC POSITIVITY

The idea that "just staying positive!" can become toxic and unhelpful. It's the practice of only focusing on the positive and "good" to the extent that you start to ignore, repress or deny the existence of negative moods, emotions or situations. Staying positive and "looking on the bright side" can be helpful, but, often, ignoring a situation is a temporary solution at best, and downright negligent and insensitive at worst.

Telling someone (yourself included) to be positive when something terrible has happened, or when they are genuinely suffering, is unhelpful. It does nothing to acknowledge the pain of the situation. Focusing on the positive in negative situations or when major issues are undeniable is a luxury and privilege most people don't have. It is wrong to believe that trying to "rewire our brain" to be more positive means ignoring anything negative, never having a negative thought or emotion again, or thinking that meditation will solve every single problem that crops up. It won't.

Often, when we pretend that a situation is better than it is, we delay the inevitable surfacing of that problem, or push it down and make it worse. As they say, "What we resist, persists." The immense pressure of pretending everything is fine, or trying to force ourselves or others to feel only positive emotions when we don't, can pile on extra pressure, making us, and those around us, feel worse in the long run. Instead, we need to *acknowledge* the situation for how it is, and work with that reality clearly.

That's why you won't ever see any Instagram posts from me saying, "Good vibes only". That's not real life.

Spiritual bypassing

That brings me to the phrase, "spiritual bypassing". The late psychotherapist John Welwood coined and defined it as, "Using spiritual ideas and practices to sidestep personal, emotional 'unfinished business,' to shore up a shaky sense of self, or to belittle basic needs, feelings, and developmental tasks."[18]

In practice, it can often look like someone sending you the message "love and light", instead of engaging in critical thought or responding to a difficult question, or questioning their own damaging behaviour and beliefs. It might be people hiding behind the words "Be kind!" to avoid debate, or saying, "Why can't we all just be nice?" when people have understandably raised their voices in anger against some injustice. It's political leaders sending "thoughts and prayers" to the victims of gun violence – instead of actively working to do something about it.

It can lead to people retreating inside their spiritual practices, treating them as a privileged and rarefied space away from anything difficult, challenging or critical... and, in the worst cases, it can enable people to continue with toxic and damaging behaviour under the cover of "spirituality". Meditation gets accused of enabling this – of encouraging people to go inwards and hide inside their own minds, selfishly, in their own bubble – rather than taking any kind of active steps to make concrete changes in the real world.

Obviously, if you're meditating *solely* for this reason, then you need to rethink why and how you're doing it, and avoid spiritual bypassing as much as possible. (More on this in Chapter 15.)

The aim is not to use meditation as a coping mechanism, like a sticking plaster over a gaping wound, without addressing the underlying cause of the problem. This will potentially cause far more harm in the long-run.

True self-compassion is when you are totally aware of what's going on – positives and negatives – and you acknowledge all the things you *do* like about yourself, and forgive yourself for all the ways you suffer, fall short, struggle, or have acted in ways you weren't proud of. Most of all, to recognize there is still so much you have to learn.

You can then give yourself the space and love you need to heal, and/or do something about it. Maybe journal it out, change a habit or behaviour, speak to a friend or a loved one, join an online support group or community, or seek help from a therapist or counsellor if necessary; rather than staying stuck, feeling as though you're the only one suffering in shame, self-loathing and fear. Because life feels a heck of a lot easier when you're on your own side.

So, how do I meditate with self-compassion in mind?

One of my favourite meditation tools to build self-compassion is "loving-kindness". Known as "metta" in Theravada Buddhism, it has existed for centuries in many traditions, but has been spearheaded in the West by the brilliant meditation teacher and co-founder of the Insight Meditation Society in Barry, Massachusetts, Sharon Salzberg.

Very simply, loving-kindness involves repeating a number of phrases to yourself as you sit in meditation, wishing yourself and others safety, wellness, happiness and ease. It may seem overly simple, but the science shows us that it actually works, and that compassion meditation is *even more fast-acting* than simple mindfulness. Studies have shown increased connectivity in brain areas for empathy and positive feelings after as little as seven hours of practice. Researchers Daniel Goleman and Richard J. Davidson have even found that "as little as two weeks of practice is sufficient to produce less mind-wandering and better focus".[19]

Sharon Salzberg famously tells a personal story of how, during a retreat, she was learning loving-kindness, but didn't feel as though it was working (a feeling familiar to meditators everywhere!). Yet, she persisted, figuring she might as well keep going until her retreat was over. One day, she knocked over a glass jar, and it smashed. To her amazement, she realized that her inner voice, rather than scolding her, was loving. Instead of barking, "You're so clumsy and useless!" at her, it said, "You're so clumsy, but I love you." She cleared up the glass and moved on with her day. She realized that, somehow, the practice had begun to percolate through her brain, and rewire her thoughts from being negative and scolding to loving and helpful.[20]

I would take the lesson learned from Sharon's anecdote further. Rather than, "You're so clumsy, *but* I love you", I would tweak it to say, "You're so clumsy, *and* I love you." Because the action may have been "negative" but that doesn't mean that *you, as a person*, are bad or negative.

Sharon has also written about an event she co-hosted with the Dalai Lama in 1989, when she told him that many Western people feel hatred toward themselves. The Dalai Lama didn't understand. In his language, Tibetan – as well as in the older languages of Sanskrit and the "Buddha's language",

Pali – there is no word for self-hatred, and he had never heard of it. He only knew the word "compassion".

As Dr Kristen Neff says, self-compassion is different to self-esteem, because it's not dependent on things going well, or on feeling better than others. She writes:

"You can't always have high self-esteem, and your life will continue to be flawed... but self-compassion will always be there, waiting for you, a safe haven... It does take work to break the self-criticising habits of a lifetime, but... it's easier than you might think, and it could change your life."[21]

MEDITATION TOOL

Loving-kindness for yourself

In a seated meditation position, close your eyes if you choose, and bring your attention to any areas of your body that feel good or pleasant. Relax into those areas and allow yourself to enjoy any feelings of warmth or softness. Breathe normally.

Hold an image of yourself in your mind, and repeat, "May I be safe, may I be happy, may I be healthy, may I feel good in my body." Repeat it at a speed that feels natural.

Change or add to the phrases, if you like, to ensure they really resonate with you. Repeat. Notice how you feel, without judgement.

5

Meditation for Anxiety

(or, How to Dial Down the Noise in your Head)

"Meditation is not a way of making your mind quiet. It is a way of entering into the quiet that is already there – buried under the 50,000 thoughts the average person thinks every day."

Deepak Chopra, author and self-help expert

So many of us live almost exclusively in our own heads. Our minds spin with stories, assumptions, fears, anxieties, regrets and future plans, chatting endlessly. It always makes me think of that phrase in *The Bell Jar* by Sylvia Plath, where she describes feeling as though she is carrying around a head "like a balloon on a string".[1] She wasn't talking about her own head – but wow, did I relate to that when I first read it. "Yes, hello, I appear to have lost my body. I am stuck in my thoughts, tethered only by a string; please help!"

Even now, almost nothing I post on Instagram gets more of a response than when I ask: "Who else here is an overthinker?". Everyone thinks they're the only one, and that everyone else's brain works rationally. Newsflash – it doesn't. They're stuck in their own stories, too.

As Anaïs Nin once quoted in 1961: "We don't see things as they are; we see them as *we* are."[2] The stories we tell ourselves about our life – what we can and cannot do, why others are acting the way they are, and why something has or has not happened to us – are playing on such a loop in our brains that we often don't even realize they're there.

Constant noise

Because we're so used to this "noise" in our minds, we think this is who we are. We take what we think as "fact". Sometimes, we are so afraid of what we might find if we "turn off" the noise – yep, you guessed it, through meditation – that we don't even want to try it. We think it must be better to be anxious, overthinking and constantly distracted, than to discover what we might find when we turn down that din.

We fear that we don't know how to fix what's underneath the noise, and that feels scarier. So, we stay stuck: scrolling, eating, drinking, distracted, replaying the past or obsessively planning the future, trying to riddle our way out of the mental mess.

A famous 2014 study by psychologist Timothy Wilson at the University of Virginia, found that a significant percentage of undergraduate students would rather give themselves an electric shock than sit quietly with their thoughts for 15 minutes (despite previously saying that they would pay to avoid being shocked).[3]

This approach can translate into severe, life-limiting anxiety, where we stay so stuck in worry and rumination that we find ourselves missing our real lives, so hung up are we on the past or future, neither of which we can control.

Facing the facts about anxiety

I am not belittling or dismissing anxiety. In fact, I know from personal experience that it can be very real, physical and terrifying. And five major anxiety disorders are officially recognized in the Diagnostic and Statistical Manual of Mental Disorders (DSM-5), used in the USA to diagnose medical mental health problems.

In the UK, the NHS recognizes generalized anxiety disorder (GAD) as an official condition, "a feeling of unease, such as worry or fear, that can be mild or severe". Crucially, it distinguishes between "perfectly normal" anxiety, such as feeling "worried and anxious about sitting an exam, or having a medical test or job interview", and people who "find it hard to control their worries", which are "more constant and can often affect their daily lives", and can mean they "struggle to remember the last time they felt relaxed."[4]

Many of us identify with the latter. I know I have. We're not alone. In June 2020, updated statistics provided by the

UK mental health charity Mind showed that as many as 8 in 100 people are being diagnosed with mixed anxiety and depression, and 6 in 100 are diagnosed with GAD, every *week*.[5] And the Mental Health Foundation asserts that, in 2013, a study found that there were 8.2 million cases of anxiety in the UK. Another study found that in England, women are almost twice as likely to be diagnosed with anxiety disorders than men.[6] In the US, research by the Center for Disease Control and Prevention (CDC) found that from August 2020 to February 2021, the percentage of adults with symptoms of an anxiety or a depressive disorder during the previous seven days increased significantly, from 36.4% to 41.5%.[7]

Sometimes, this anxiety is a natural response to stress, and can be solved by being a bit kinder to ourselves – taking a break, saying "no" more, planning better, and cancelling commitments. But, often, we may find that we wake up anxious for no reason, and the slightest thing can make us feel desperate and unsafe. Our brains may start to jump from one thing to the next until we're panicking.

As my Buddhist teacher Lodro Rinzler always reminds me, an anxious mind easily extrapolates a small problem to a bigger one, and then a bigger one, over and over, until pretty soon we imagine we'll surely lose everything, and end up living in a cardboard box under a bridge, feeling like an utter failure with no friends. One of my all-time favourite researchers and writers on shame and vulnerability, Brené Brown, has referred to this sort of thinking as "catastrophizing". It means we imagine the most catastrophic outcome, or tell ourselves that something bad *must* be about to happen, when things are going "too" well.

This is basically our brain trying to keep us safe. We think that if we pre-empt all possible worries, and consider all possible outcomes before they happen, we'll be protected if or when something terrible does happen. But the research shows that, in many cases, this catastrophizing and worrying doesn't help. It just makes us more anxious, and therefore, arguably, less likely to cope if the worst does happen. And, usually, we're doing so much better than we think we are.

Anxiety as identity

Many of us might think we *need* to worry – especially if we see ourselves as having a "type A", organized personality. We might believe that our anxiety helps us to stay vigilant, alert and on top of things. After all, we think, if we don't worry about getting to places on time, then won't we be late and miss everything?

When we're generally a high-alert, anxious sort of person, we might almost take *pride* in our worry. We feel that we're more realistic or "switched on" than other people, who seem to stumble around in blissful ignorance, blithely missing trains and losing passports with abandon. It can be *infuriating* to be someone who feels like you *have to* worry. If *we* don't worry and keep track, then *who will*?

But studies have shown that after a certain point – beyond a sensible amount of preparation, worrying about the future doesn't make us more resilient or likely to cope with disaster. In fact, a 2015 study found that young people who tended toward catastrophizing-style thought patterns were more likely to have anxiety disorders;[8] while a 2012 study found that an anxious state of mind could even *cause depression,* because "assuming that the worst will always happen leads to feelings of hopelessness",[9] which is really not great for our mental health.

It's clear that anxiety and overthinking are inextricably linked. A 2012 review of studies found that catastrophizing could even make *fatigue* worse – coming as no surprise to anyone who's ever spent hours overthinking something endlessly.[10] Of course, depression is complex and has many causes – biological, physiological and social – but for the purposes of this chapter, the science does bear out the Randy Armstrong quote: "Worrying does not take away tomorrow's troubles. It takes away today's peace." Long story short, anxiety doesn't help us plan better. It just makes us less productive and more worried.

So, how can we change this? How do we get to that place of self-awareness and self-compassion where we recognize that we're caught in overthinking, and give ourselves permission to stop and rest? If we're someone who has been living in an overthinking, anxious mind for years – and it's all we know – how can meditation and mindfulness help us?

How mindfulness helps

1. It gives us mental space
Learning to come back to the present through meditation doesn't mean we never think about the past or future, or consider

how we could have handled something differently. It just means that we're no longer obsessing about it; we can look at it in a more level-headed way, with compassion and clear-headedness, instead of getting stuck in anxiety.

We know that we can come back to the clarity that the present offers us, and that we're safe, grounded and supported in our current moment, no matter what. The more we practise, the more we notice the thoughts we're having *before* we get sucked in, and learn to ask simple questions that stop them in their tracks, such as:

- Is this worrying helpful?
- Is this train of thought helping me to make a better decision?
- Is worrying about my work going to help me plan better or do better?
- Am I channelling this worry into productive, useful action?
- And once I've planned that action or done that thing, am I going to drop this worry, and get on with my life, secure in the knowledge that I've done everything I can?

If yes, *genuinely*, then carry on. But, if not – we can ask ourselves:

- Is this train of thought unhelpful?
- Is it damaging or useless?
- Am I just ruminating or worrying about things I can't control?

2. It interrupts thinking

Here's the thing: we can't think our way out of thinking. If we could, we'd have done it by now.

And it's a cliché, but has a kernel of truth: The only thing we have is the present moment – our body, right here, right now. As frustrating as this can sound, if we sit with it and feel it in our bones, it can be very reassuring. "Forever is composed of nows",[11] the poet Emily Dickinson once wrote. So if, in each "now", we can learn how to feel safe in our bodies in the present, we're learning how to get through almost anything, one breath at a time.

I'm not saying it's easy. It isn't. It can be one of the hardest and scariest things to learn if you struggle with anxiety and panic – especially if it's as a result of trauma. But it's possible, through gentle, sustained practice.

Learning how to feel safe in ourselves, focus our mind through the power of the breath, and use it to connect and get grounded through our physical body, is one of *the* most powerful tools we have for interrupting anxiety, panic, overthinking and overwhelm. It enables us to feel secure and solid in the here, the now, and the present, exactly as we are.

The myth of clearing your mind

A crucial point: "interrupting thinking" when meditating doesn't mean we're aiming to "think of nothing".

As Dan Harris of podcast 10% Happier has said, "Clearing your mind is impossible, unless you're enlightened or dead."[12] Trying to make our mind go blank is not the goal. The goal is to readjust its focus – to guide it toward something more present, solid and real – rather than allowing our focus to spiral out of control, conjecturing about the past or the future.

As Timothy Wilson, the psychologist who did the electric shock study I referred to earlier, told the scientific journal *Science* in 2014, "I think [our] mind is built to engage in the world. So, when we don't give it anything to focus on, it's kind of hard to know what to do."[13]

We're also learning how to go *beyond* our busy minds, and send our attention into our physical body. In fact, this is about stopping seeing the mind and body as separate at all. That's why mindfulness teachers will always ask you to not just notice the breath, but also *where* in the body you can feel it. That's what I mean by "being in the body" as a different way to experience the world, beyond our minds, thoughts and even language. The part of our brain that goes online when we do this is called the insular cortex (or "the insula"). It's what we're using when we feel our own heartbeat, for example.

Being mindful and learning to meditate is also about understanding that everything we think and feel has a mirror effect in our physical body, and vice-versa. As Bessel A. van der Kolk, psychologist and author of the book *The Body Keeps The Score* says, "In order to change, people need to become aware of their sensations and the way that their bodies interact with the world around them."[14]

To go back to *The Bell Jar* analogy: We are not just balloons on a string. We are human beings, with living, breathing and feeling bodies and minds, and the two are inextricably linked. This may seem a weird concept if you've never come across it before. And yet, in many ways, it's totally normal. We talk about getting "butterflies in our stomach" when we feel nervous. We might blush if we think something embarrassing, or feel sick when we remember something we forgot to do.

Anxiety shows up in exactly the same way. As anyone with anxiety knows, it has as many physical symptoms as mental ones – including shakes, headaches, stomach aches and nausea. In fact, once you tune in to your physical body and mind, you may start to notice stress in your body long before you might otherwise think you need to take a break. Our bodies offer an incredibly sensitive set of extra tools for interpreting the world, and we can use them to build a new relationship with ourselves in the process.

This in itself can be revolutionary for women. So many of us were taught that our minds were the most important thing. Our grades, our intellectual work, our ability to reason, write and articulate, was vital. And, unless we were a sports prodigy, it's unlikely that as kids our physical ability was prized anywhere near as much as that of boys. So many of us were told that if we worked a little harder, thought a little more, studied a little longer, we would know the answer. And in some ways, sure, that works. But, in truth, the magazine article that kickstarted my interest in meditation, entitled "Think Yourself Happy", only told *half* the story – meditation isn't just about *thinking* yourself happy, it's about *feeling* your way to "happy", too.

Meditation gives you the tools to regulate your mind, breath *and* body. It gives you permission to open up that two-way connection between your body and your brain, which may have become blocked without you even knowing.

Another word on trauma

As I said earlier, I do not mean to offer meditation as a magic panacea, nor to downplay how terrible anxiety can be. There are certainly types of anxiety and mental distress that require even more care, and those that cause extreme physical reactions, such as post-traumatic stress disorder (PTSD), which is one of the kinds of anxiety specifically recognised by the DSM-5.

After a traumatic event, it's perfectly normal to experience stress in a million different ways, and it can be your body's way of coping. The only issue is that, if we don't eventually deal with this trauma response, it can keep us stuck and scared, and even more traumatized. As I explained in the last chapter, trauma comes in many forms, and it's important to be aware of it when meditating. Most people will be able to meditate without issues, but some may find that it can increase distress if not done with care.

Mindful trauma specialist David A. Treleaven describes a "window of tolerance".[15] Think of your mental space as a split sponge cake, with icing in the middle (the cake metaphor is mine, sorry David). Mentally, we're aiming for the middle, sitting in that icing layer between the two halves of the cake: neither too "high" nor too "low".

That "middle" is where we can use mindfulness to "come home" to our body, and feel safe. If we go too "high", our minds feel stressed and we might dissociate from our surroundings, trying to escape; we may "check out", with physical symptoms such as a racing heart or sweating profusely, wanting to escape to anywhere but here. If we go too "low", we may close in on ourselves, slow down, get sluggish and distracted, and "check out" in a lethargic way, unable to focus, feeling exhausted and even depressed.

Both are understandable ways to escape the situation, find relief from trauma, stress and anxiety. But neither is sustainable. Regular and compassionate mindfulness practice can guide us to a mental and physical state in which we feel calm and safe enough to be with ourselves, without retraumatizing ourselves. We can instead retreat safely into the body and breath to find relief from stress.

Don't sweat the small stuff

For many of us, however, stress isn't caused by trauma – at least, not all the time. It's caused by the bullshit of everyday life, with its tiny irritations and stupid arguments, incompetence, bureaucracy, and the sheer mundanity of everyday adult responsibility. As Jean-Paul Sartre said: "Hell is other people."[16]

Sometimes, stress and anxiety are caused by having too much to do, not enough time to do it in, and the endless disappointment of things never being as easy as you think they should be. But you know that phrase: "Don't sweat the small stuff (and it's all small stuff)"? Well, meditation helps us to put that into practice.

Recently, I had one of *those* days, where everything takes 20% longer than you anticipated, you woke up later than you meant to and it feels like you're wearing an itchy jumper that's half a size too small. My bank accidentally cancelled all my cards,

I missed an important call from my doctor, and there were a million other tiny, stupid things. It was a mess. A few years ago, this kind of day would have finished me off emotionally. My inner critic would have been *deafening*: "You should be better prepared. You always do this. You're such a failure; everyone else has their shit together except you." On and on she would have gone, making everything feel a million times worse.

But with mindfulness, we can get perspective on all that noise and negativity. The voice might not stop, but we can change it from vicious to helpful. We can draw a line under the bad day, and try again tomorrow. Maybe we can even check our schedule and learn what, if anything, we can learn from the crappy day when we try to do better tomorrow.

Mindfulness helps us to separate negative situations from feeling negative about ourselves as a human. We are still worthy, even on our worst days. Employing the tools of mindfulness allows us to take a break from the stories in our head, and stop making one small thing mean something about who we are as a human. It helps us to keep things in perspective – sometimes, a bad day is just a bad day. It doesn't mean you're a bad person with a shit life.

This is not because mindfulness turns us all into passive saints who never get caught up in the little things. It's because mindfulness teaches us how to zoom out, refocus and remember what's important to us. We can ask: "Do I really want to give my energy to this?"

It's like that quote: "If it costs you your peace, it's too expensive." And I am no longer prepared to pay for all this bullshit to live rent-free in my head. Meditation teaches us that we are of value, even if we fuck up. Even if we have a totally chaotic "one of those days", or something crappy happens, we still matter. We can learn from it, and then move on – perhaps mildly annoyed, but not with so much pent-up anger than it ruins our whole day.

Stop the story

This "acceptance" – one of the key tenets of mindfulness and meditation – is simply about seeing what *is*, without judgement, and not getting stuck in a loop of anxiety or overthinking. It can also give us the space we need to be grateful for what is going well, even if we have had a total shitshow of a day.

As the meditation expert Professor Mark Williams often says, mindfulness can be a great thing to practise when we're stuck in traffic, or in a queue.[17] It's annoying, but there's not a lot we can do about it, and getting stressed won't fix or improve it, so we may as well relax. What else can we focus on instead? The fact that everyone is safe? The surprisingly beautiful colour of the autumn leaves? That at least we're healthy enough to stand in the queue, or that we can afford a car in which to sit in traffic?

It's a small mindset tweak. It doesn't make the frustration go away, but it allows us to *sit with whatever is,* and not tell ourselves a whole fabricated story, or jump to conclusions. Mindfulness allows us to accept ourselves and the situation, as they are. And in a world that can present us with no end of irritating, shitty small stuff, that can be of great consolation.

MEDITATION TOOL

Ocean breath

Once seated in meditation, close your eyes if you feel comfortable. Notice your body sitting: the texture of the chair, the feeling of gravity. Drop your shoulders and relax the skin of your face.

Notice what you can hear, feel, smell or taste.

Now bring your attention to your breath. Is it shallow or deep?

Try to slow your breathing if you can. Inhale through your nose for a count of three, and exhale out of your mouth for a count of four. Allow your lungs to expand fully as you inhale, and allow your muscles to relax and "melt" into the chair as you exhale. You might imagine your breath like an ocean, inhaling as the "waves" come in, exhaling as the "waves" go out.

When you get distracted, come back to it and begin again, noticing the breath and your entire body.

Repeat for as long as you need.

6

Working through Heartbreak and Grief

(or, Meditating when Life's Even Tougher than Usual)

"We all experience heartbreak. It might be personal, such as a break-up, sure, but it might also stem from job loss, the death of a loved one, or just not feeling like we're living up to our potential."

Lodro Rinzler, author and meditation teacher

Let's be real: some stuff in life isn't small. Some stuff is pretty fucking huge. Massive life transitions, terminal diagnoses, death, life-altering injuries or illnesses, heartbreak, major disappointment, financial stress, abuse, severe mental illness... these are not challenges we can just shrug off.

You're grieving, for all of it – for anything in life that breaks your heart. Anything that isn't living up to how we believe it should be or want it to be can cause us to feel this way, whether that's our career, our relationship, wider global issues, our parents, our job, or even how we view ourselves and what we see as our own (lack of) success.

A particularly apt wordplay lyric from Taylor's Swift's "lockdown" album *Folklore* describes this feeling perfectly: "They told me all of my cages were mental, so I got wasted like all my potential."[1] If that doesn't describe how life can feel sometimes, then I don't know what to tell you.

Luckily, in his TEDx talk, entrepreneur and researcher into the economics of happiness, Nat Ware, offers us a helpful way to consider this. He calls it the "expectation gap" – the difference between where we are, and where we think we should be.[2] It's my belief that so much unhappiness in life comes from this exact space. And it can easily feel like one ginormous, impossible-to-bridge abyss, and a source of deep suffering.

Life transitions

It's of absolutely no surprise to me that around 90% of my clients sign up to work with me during times of major life transition, whether that's a new job, a career change, a break-up or divorce, a work challenge, following an accident or diagnosis, or ahead of an imminent cross-country move. They are consistently looking for support as they navigate these significant changes and take their next steps.

I now think of these major life experiences as "lifequakes" – a term I learned from the *New York Times* bestselling author Bruce Feiler, who coins it in his most recent book, *Life Is In the Transitions: Mastering Change in a Nonlinear Age.*[3]

As the book's title suggests, he states that throughout our lives we all experience events that are "lifequakes" – major transitions, both good and bad. They tend to be events that cause us to think of life "before" and "after" that event, and they each add different – perhaps unexpected – chapters to our overall story. The book explains that we are often defined by the story we tell ourselves about our lives, and we also tend to expect our lives to run in a linear fashion – like a neat, upwards line graph on a blank piece of paper. We think that we need to get from A to B to C – from school to a job to marriage, for example – and we also may imagine that the path there will be largely straightforward. If this happens, we feel that our lives are, in Feiler's own words, "ascending" – on the up.

But any deviation from that – a serious diagnosis, a death of a loved one, a major break-up, a career-changing mistake or pivot – throws a spanner in the works. These "lifequakes", which take us away from that neat, linear narrative we believed our life would follow, can cause us to feel heartbreak, as life isn't panning out the way we intended. Our happiness, or lack thereof, can be traced back to the nice straight line that we thought our life would draw, compared to the jumbled scrawl we feel it's actually scribbling.

But the answer is not to lower our expectations or resort to the platitude that "everything happens for a reason". Saying that doesn't exactly make difficult times any easier, does it? I find it more helpful to remember that the late Swiss psychiatrist Elisabeth Kübler-Ross first defined her now-famous "five stages of grief"[4]: denial, anger, bargaining, depression and, finally, acceptance. When tragedy strikes, we might immediately begin going through these stages without even realizing, and it can feel unnerving as heck to find ourselves an unwilling passenger on this rollercoaster of emotion.

Not only that, but Kübler-Ross herself was keen to point out that the "stages" aren't linear. We don't jump through them like hoops, but cycle through them randomly, feeling anger on one day, depression on another, and back to denial again the next week. Healing isn't linear – just as our lives aren't. No wonder heartbreak can feel like the world's crappiest rollercoaster.

Interestingly, Kübler-Ross's former co-worker, grief expert David Kessler, recently added an extra stage to the "five stages" in his 2019 book *Finding Meaning: The Sixth Stage of Grief* [5] – as the title suggests, the sixth stage was "meaning".

As Kessler explained in a viral article with the *Harvard Business Review*, "I did not want to stop at acceptance when I experienced some personal grief [the death of his son]. I wanted meaning in those darkest hours. And I do believe we can find light in those times." [6]

That didn't make what happened OK, and Kessler himself has said that he still wishes – it almost goes without saying – that his son hadn't passed away. But finding meaning, he said, was some comfort.

Mindfulness and mourning

When heartbreak or tragedy hits, it can be a massive relief to have an anchor to hold on to in those stormy emotional seas. Something keeping us grounded, allowing us to come back to ourselves, to feel a modicum of comfort and reassurance, even if everything feels utterly shit, is important. Mindfulness, meditation and self-compassion can be that anchor. As Kessler said:

> "To calm yourself, you want to come into the present. This will be familiar advice to anyone who has meditated or practiced mindfulness... [but] it's that simple... You can also think about how to let go of what you can't control... [Now] is a good time to stock up on compassion."[7]

Indeed, for me, at the lowest and most confusing times in my life – after a horrendous break-up, when someone I love was diagnosed with cancer, when my dad was in hospital after a sudden heart attack, when depression led me to believe that my life wasn't worth living and that I was a total waste of space – meditation has been there, waiting for me, welcoming me into its accepting, non-judgemental arms, saying, "I know things feel utterly broken right now, and you don't know what to do, or how to fix it. But that's OK, because you are safe here. Your meditation practice is a haven. It's OK to be who you are, even if life is awful right now. Let it out. Sit. Breathe. Repair. Rebuild."

Meditation is not about sweeping terrible things under the rug, pretending we're OK and carrying on. It's the opposite. It's about building the courage and steadfastness within ourselves to *turn toward* the pain and suffering we feel, forgive ourselves for it, investigate how it feels, and know that we have a safe foundation within our own mind to come back to or escape to, no matter what. It shows us how to build a safe and kind space inside our head when the world around us feels anything but.

As the wise (and funny) Buddhist nun Pema Chödrön writes in her classic book *When Things Fall Apart*:

> *"We think that the point is to pass the test or overcome the problem, but the truth is that things don't really get solved. They come together and they fall apart... The healing comes from letting there be room for all of this to happen: room for grief, for relief, for misery, for joy."*[8]

It's about being kind to yourself and realizing that you are not alone in your suffering, that others have suffered like this before you, and that perhaps it might be time for you to reach out – call a friend, or consult a grief counsellor or professional therapist to help you process and work through your emotions.

Mindfulness is not about forcing yourself to shoulder burdens alone because of how "calm" your mind is, or how much work you've put into your practice. Asking for help and getting therapy, or taking anti-anxiety or anti-depressant medication if you and your doctor agree you need it, is fine too. I've personally done both during hard times, and they acted as an excellent complement to my meditation in getting my mental health back on track.

Mindfulness is about recognizing how you feel, forgiving yourself for it, and then choosing a compassionate path for yourself by identifying what you need and what will help you feel better in the long-run (and not through self-destructive options such as excessive food, booze or drugs). Building compassion and acceptance in the face of tragedy doesn't make the impossible, unthinkable, terrible things go away... but it does help get you away from the edge of the metaphorical cliff, and get your mind back to a place where you feel a tiny bit more able to confront things and breathe. It can offer you the space you need to just be, to regroup and to allow yourself to get through whatever pain and suffering you're experiencing.

Mindful moments

Meditation trains us to use our five senses, and remembering this during a time of grief and heartbreak particularly can help. Noticing tastes, sights, smells and feelings can – perhaps bizarrely – help us soothe the pain inside our heart and mind. As Kessler says:

"People are always surprised at how prosaic this can be... Breathe... In this moment, you're okay... Use your senses and think about what they feel. The desk is hard. The blanket is soft. I can feel the breath coming into my nose. This really will work to dampen some of that pain."[9]

Personally, after one particularly bad break-up, I used to start every single day by listening to the song *"New York Morning"* by the band Elbow.[10] For some reason, that song lifted me right out of my funk. I could somehow feel it travelling from my ears, resonating down my shoulders and arms and rippling like ocean waves in my fingers. Through these sensations, I let it carry my mind away – if not necessarily *happier* things, then definitely further away from the weight of my sad, broken heart. Noticing those physical sensations saved me. I still get chills when I hear the song now, as I am reminded of that optimism, which seemed to come from nowhere, even at a very low moment in my life.

During other terrible times, I've found great solace in mindfully walking, noticing the way the sun reflects on the surface of a river, the deep blue colour of the sky, or the sounds of birds singing. That may sound trite and obvious, but I don't give a crap, because that stuff truly helps me. Just as I've wondered how the world can possibly continue to keep turning when everything in my own world feels as though it's imploding, the small part of my mind that is able to remain mindful and sensitive to sights and sounds finds a tiny spark of hope in these little moments.

Of course, they don't make heartbreak or grief OK. But to remember that birds will sing and the sun will come up tomorrow, can offer a tiny, tiny reminder that this too will pass, and that just as the world keeps turning, you will one day feel a bit better. Sometimes the hope of that alone is enough to get you through another day.

Change is constant

Mindfulness principles help us to accept these most painful parts of life, too. As I first heard from the insight meditation teacher and leadership coach Anushka Fernandopulle, we can consider the concept of change as we consider gravity.[11] Gravity is always there; it's constant. We don't question it, or make it personal. If gravity pulls us down, we don't think it's because we've done something wrong, that we are undeserving. It's just the way things are. We can't fight it. The only thing we can do is accept it, concede to it, and make the best of our life knowing that we cannot change it.

In the same way, it's a solid Buddhist principle to remember that everything in life changes. It may seem nihilistic and morbid to contemplate, but everything living will one day die.

Just as the leaves fall and die in autumn, it can be remarkably peaceful to see that things ending and breaking down are all part and parcel of what it means to live in an ever-changing world as a human being. This doesn't make everything OK, but it can, in some cases, take the edge off our pain, and our concerns about others, alleviating the feeling that we are uniquely alone in our suffering, and allowing us to continue living through it, breath by breath.

Helping others through grief or heartbreak

These principles can also help us to help others. We can recognize that we're all human and that, one day, we might be experiencing something similar to what this person is going through right now. Shifting perspective in this way helps us to think of others compassionately, and send them kind and loving thoughts and actions. If someone we know is ill and suffering, say, or a relative is dealing with terrible news, we often want to empathize with their pain, even if we don't know what to say. Learning to sit with our own suffering without instantly rushing to fix it, teaches us how to do the same with others, too.

We can sit with someone in their grief and recognize it as a normal (if terrible) part of the human experience, and not feel utterly uncomfortable. Just sitting with someone who is in pain, even in silence – as we learn to do with ourselves through meditation – can be incredibly helpful to them.

Just as we might feel like a burden to others when we are suffering, other people might fear they are being a burden to us; it can be powerful to realize that they have a friend who is not going to run, or resort to suggesting "solutions" at the first sign of pain or trouble. And, as that friend, we may feel as though we are, in our own small way, helping.

Insight through pain

Lastly, sometimes feelings of heartbreak and grief can be signposts to wake us up to a situation that isn't working for us anymore. Just as feeling jealous or comparing ourselves negatively to someone can be seen as a "crystal of insight" as to what we're really feeling, as the Comparison Coach Lucy Sheridan puts it,[12] so pain and grief can lead us to gather the courage we need to change a bad situation.

As horrendous as it is, heartbreak or "hitting rock bottom" can be one heck of a catalyst. For example, it might show us that we need to leave a toxic or abusive situation, quit a job we hate, or change major parts of our life, even if that's terrifying. This is where building a safe, kind and welcoming space within our minds and bodies helps. The idea that we can go back there whenever we need to can be incredibly reassuring. No matter what life holds, if we know that we're on our own side no matter what, we may feel less alone, less broken, and find the strength to keep going. And maybe – just maybe – we'll find happiness again, too.

MEDITATION TOOL

Breathing through emotional pain

In a comfortable position, close your eyes if you like. Breathe as deeply as you can, slowing down your breath. Let your exhales be longer than your inhales.

Gently and kindly, notice any painful thoughts, or how your grief is showing up physically. Where can you feel it in your body? Tense, tight, hot, heavy, tearful, numb... there are no wrong answers. It's OK to find this painful and difficult. At any time, remember that you can stop. Hold yourself in a hug, or hold a comforting object, if it helps.

As you inhale, imagine your body is hollow, like a blown egg, and "send" your new breath to the areas where you feel that grief. Allow the oxygen to "air" those spaces out, and bring space to the tightness or pain.

As you exhale, allow your muscles to relax and deflate, noticing your body is secure, safe and grounded. Notice what, if anything, changes.

Repeat.

7

Meditation for Owning It

(or, Giving Fewer Shits about What Other People Think)

"Do you know how old you will be by the time I learn to really play the piano / act / paint / write a decent play? Yes... the same age you will be if you don't."

Julia Cameron, *The Artist's Way*

Doing your own thing in life can be terrifying. If you're someone with big dreams, you're probably going against the norm, doing things people don't expect from you, trying something new and untested, or something less secure than your current path. It's easy to self-sabotage before you even start because you're so afraid of what others think, or too busy trying to get their approval.

This is when meditation – ultimately, the practice of getting to know yourself underneath all the external noise – is key. When you know your own path, you can turn down the dial on other people's judgement, stop waiting for approval, and do whatever the heck you want. It's like that Charles Bukowski quote: "Remember who you were before the world told you who to be."

When I first started my business, I craved approval and support from everyone I knew. I wanted everybody to be my loudest supporters, give me all the business advice, "like" every single one of my social posts, be there at every online and IRL event, recommend me to their friends, write about me in all their journalistic pieces on wellbeing, and refer my business to everyone they met.

When that didn't happen, I was stung. I felt like I'd supported them when they'd had terrible jobs, got new ones, suffered through bad relationships, adopted pets, got married, moved house, had kids, and all the rest of it. And yet, when it was my turn to do something that felt momentous to me, I was met with confusion, a few rude questions, and jokes – but mainly, a whole load of silence.

Some people were supportive, but others told me straight up that I was making a mistake and should have stayed doing what I was doing before. People openly laughed when I told them why I was leaving my 9-to-5. Even now, people ask, "Are you still doing that meditation thing?" and "Is meditation something people even, like, *need*?". They question, still, whether I can possibly help anyone, because I don't have a PhD in psychiatry, and suggest that I've "wasted my education" by doing something slightly more creative than becoming a management consultant.

I'm not necessarily blaming them. It's society's fault, really, for suggesting that we should all aspire to a life path and job title that doesn't cause blank stares and awkward silences at dinner parties.

But this isn't a "poor me" story, despite what it might sound like. Because the thing is, despite what society and our own brains tell us, *it actually doesn't matter what other people think or do.*

But first, let's check: Is comparison (negative and/or positive) an issue for you?

COMPARISON SPIRAL QUIZ

Answer yes/no and count up the number of yes answers.

1. Do you often find yourself feeling worse rather than better after time on social media? Y/N
2. Do you ever feel like nothing you do is good enough, because someone/others out there are already doing it better? Y/N
3. Do you ever feel like you could work all the hours of the day, but it would never be enough? Y/N
4. Do you find yourself doing or buying things simply to post about it / tell others? Y/N
5. If I ask you to think of someone whose life makes you feel bad about your own, does someone (or multiple people) immediately spring to mind? Y/N
6. If someone announces a big life event (engagement, baby, dream job) is your first reaction to feel bad about yourself, or feel anger or pain, because you haven't done the same thing? Y/N
7. Do you often find yourself thinking or saying that other people don't deserve their success? Y/N

8. Do you often look at others and wonder what they have that you don't? Y/N
9. Do you find yourself saying no to events / invitations because you're afraid of what other people will think of you (or that you won't feel good enough) when you're there? Y/N
10. Do you ever find yourself thinking, "Well, at LEAST I'm doing better than HER/him/them?" Y/N

How many did you get?
1–3: Caught off-balance
4–7: In a twist
8–10: Full-blown spiral

The real truth is, most people are too busy with their own lives to care much about yours, and if you wait for other people's approval or support before you believe in yourself or do what you want, then you're going to be waiting a heck of a long time.

Doing your own thing is about *you*, building up your own sense of self-confidence, regardless of what anyone else is doing, or isn't. That doesn't mean you stop caring about what others are doing… it just means you stop comparing yourself to them, measuring yourself by someone else's imagined ruler, or judging people by "achievements" at all.

The world doesn't make this easy, though. It's still incredibly frustrating that quitting the 9-to-5, starting your own business, going freelance, travelling the world, deciding not to get married or have kids, and/or making your own rules in life is still seen by many as a slightly subversive thing to do, and not particularly celebrated.

It's frustrating, and not a little weird, because it's not exactly uncommon. A study by The Federation of Small Businesses (FSB) found that there were 5.9 million small businesses in the UK at the start of 2020.[1] Similarly, a survey by business credit brokerage SME Loans found that one in three employees dislike their job, one in three would welcome flexible working and the ability to work remotely, 64% of the UK workforce wants to set up a business, and as many as 83% of 18–24-year-olds dream of self-employment.[2]

Similarly, in the US, the Small Business Administration (SBA) states that in 2019, there were 30.7 million small businesses (of which 89% had 1–20 employees), and founders' main motivations for doing their own thing was a desire to "be their own boss" (55%), and "pursue their passion" (39%).[3] The Association of Independent Professionals & the Self-Employed (IPSE) found that in 2021, in the UK, more than 4.8 million people identified as self-employed, and that a similar number of independent workers in the US now describe themselves as "digital nomads" (people who work remotely while travelling).[4]

That's a heck of a lot of people wanting to do their own thing.

And as the success of Emma Gannon's book *The Multi-Hyphen Method: Work Less, Create More: How to Make Your Side Hustle Work For You*[5] shows, starting a side hustle, and describing yourself as having more than one job title, is rapidly becoming more normal. "Doing your own thing" is pretty common these days. Despite this, many of us stay trapped, and spend years being terrified of what others think, to the point where we do nothing.

And yet, other people are probably not even thinking of us at all. At first, that may feel kinda sad, as if "no-one cares". Later, it feels absolutely freeing. But this lack of overwhelming support for different choices at the beginning of our journey can keep us small, scared, stuck and self-sabotaging, because we're so afraid of what others think. We can let one negative comment stop us in our tracks for months.

When it comes to starting businesses in particular, you won't be surprised to hear that women and minorities are more likely to hold themselves back than white men, with figures from business website Startups showing that, in 2019, only 14% of UK entrepreneurs were women, and just 7% were from an ethnic minority.[6] SME Loans found that, while "men worry more about competition and failure… women worry about not feeling qualified enough or having the relevant skills".[7]

It's no surprise to me that women are far more afraid of not being good enough – and being judged as a result. So often, we're socialized to people-please – to work hard and keep our heads down, and to follow the "job-engaged-married-kids" path – that we actually *do* feel judgement from around us if we dare to try something different. But I've learned that people will judge, misunderstand and ignore, no matter what you do, so you might as well do whatever you like. After all, it's your career, your business, your life. We can make ourselves utterly miserable in a prison of our own mind, entirely constructed by what we *think* other people might be thinking. I'm exhausted even writing this!

Personally, I know that if I'd stayed in my old job – despite it making me sick with misery – people would still have judged me. I could have bent over backwards trying to be what I thought

I was supposed to be, and it wouldn't have made any difference. It's only when you learn to let go of what other people think of you by building a rock-solid, quietly-confident inner sense of self-worth, that you feel truly free to continue in whatever you're doing. Meditation teaches us that.

The "right kind" of feedback

It's your party, and you don't want people there who pick at the food, bitch about the music, and make rude comments about your outfit bringing down the vibe. You want people who are ready to dance the house down and clink Champagne glasses when you tell them good news or, even better, who'll give you a massive hug when you share how damn difficult it's been lately.

Of course, there's a difference between unsolicited comments and constructive criticism from people who care about you and who know what they're talking about. Distinguishing between these two can be hard. That's why doing your own thing in life requires you to have an incredibly strong sense of self. You need an internal compass about who you are, where you're going, and why, and a thick skin to buffer any well-intentioned – or not so-well-intentioned – "feedback" (as the glorious Hannah Gadsby termed it in her 2018 stage show, Nanette[8]).

Ultimately, this is about setting healthy boundaries. And this is where meditation and mindfulness come in – because to set boundaries, we need self-knowledge. We need to be able to sit with ourselves, decide who and what we are and are not, and build the confidence to ensure that anyone who doesn't get it, doesn't get a say.

You don't want to harden your heart so much that you become bitter and closed off to constructive criticism and discussion; you just want to partition off certain parts of your heart to those who haven't earned the right to be there. As Brené Brown says: "Strong back, soft front, wild heart." [9]

Badass boundaries: No more people pleasing

I've also learned that when you're starting out on a new project, you do not have to be 100% honest with everyone who asks about it or who offers an opinion. You don't owe anyone anything – especially if their comments make you feel judged, mocked or unsafe. You *can* keep your distance mentally.

When we're working on something dear to our heart, we can often feel as though we have to discuss it all, to share the ups and downs, and to get others on board so they "truly understand our creative process". But we don't have to if we don't want to. As the Comparison Coach Lucy Sheridan says, sometimes the best thing to do – at least at first – is to protect your new project. Don't tell anyone, or just tell a select few people. When you're working on something new and fragile, it can take one negative comment to crush it. So don't let it. [10]

Boundaries and living mindfully aren't about forcing others to think how you do. They're just about building a strong sense of your own worth, and your own sense of what's acceptable (or not), and calmly letting others know what that is. As they say: "The only people who get upset when you set boundaries are the people who benefitted from you having none."

Here are some great comebacks I can recommend if and when people start questioning your business/life choices or offering unsolicited feedback. Take a deep breath, mindfully feel your feet to ground yourself, remind yourself why you're doing this, tell yourself that you're a badass – and calmly proceed.

- It's going well, thanks. I appreciate you asking!
  How are you?
- Yes, all good. How's *your* career/love life/job/house/book going?
- I'd prefer not to talk about that right now; I'm having a day off. How are you?
- I know you don't see eye-to-eye with me on this, so can we agree to disagree and talk about something else?
- Can you explain why you think that? That isn't my experience.
- Here's why I find that offensive/wrong/misguided/unhelpful.
- I'd love to chat with you if you have any constructive advice, but otherwise let's talk about something else.
- If you're not able to respect my choices/views on this, then I'll have to ask that we stop talking/I leave/you leave.

Basically, whenever you feel like someone is overstepping your boundaries, or talking about something that makes you feel uncomfortable, or you consider to be unfair or unkind, you are *allowed* to not respond or to ask them to stop. Don't get me wrong – this can be *really* tough, for women especially, because we're socialized to be polite and people-pleasing.

But as Florence Given, author of the book *Women Don't Owe You Pretty*, says, "When you have lived a life of people-pleasing, saying your true desires will make you feel guilty. Push through and communicate them. You didn't come here to be liked."[11]

If you want to hack your own path, work to let go of your need to be liked or approved of, and your desire to meet others' expectations.

As the Toni Morrison quote goes, "You wanna fly, you got to give up the shit that weighs you down."[12]

PEOPLE ON PAPER

A great exercise to figure out who to listen to is this:

On a small piece of paper, write down the names of maybe three to five people in your life whose opinions you really care about, but no more than that. If anyone else offers an opinion that seems hurtful or unhelpful, check if their name is on the list.

No? No opinion. Carry on.

In her excellent book *Daring Greatly*, Brené Brown also references the famous speech known as *The Man in the Arena*, by President Theodore Roosevelt. The pertinent part of the speech is:

"It is not the critic who counts; not the man who points out how the strong man stumbles, or where the doer of deeds could have done them better.

"The credit belongs to the man who is actually in the arena, whose face is marred by dust and sweat and blood; who strives valiantly; who errs, who comes short again and again, because there is no effort without error and shortcoming; but who does actually strive to do the deeds; who knows great enthusiasms, the great devotions; who spends himself in a worthy cause; who at the best knows in the end the triumph of high achievement, and who at the worst, if he fails, at least fails while daring greatly."

Brené was hugely inspired by that speech, leading her to name her book after it, and write (and repeat on stage forever after) the immortal line: "If you're not in the arena also getting your ass kicked, I'm not interested in your feedback."[13]

Opinions from people who aren't in your space, and who haven't themselves tried or done what you are trying to do? No. If it's good enough for Brené, it's good enough for us.

How meditation helps

Regular meditation helps us to develop our sense of self and intuition, so we stop *pretending* not to care what random people think and start *genuinely* not caring. Unsurprisingly, this comes from self-compassion (see Chapter 4) and forgiving yourself for all the ways you're not yet strong enough not to care what others think. Because, paradoxically, it's *normal* to care what others think. It would be quite psychopathic not to care *at all*. To use the classic example: when we were cavemen in tribes, if we tried to "go our own way", it wouldn't be long before we were eaten by a passing mammoth.

The need for connection and social approval is wired into our DNA, so we needn't beat ourselves up for it. We all need approval and to feel as though we belong to a group in some way. Matthew D. Lieberman, a professor of psychology at UCLA and the author of *Social: Why Our Brains Are Wired to Connect*, once told the *New York Times* that our need for positive social interaction "has been there in one form or another since before the dinosaurs 250 million years ago".[14]

In his research, Dr Lieberman monitored the brains of people playing a video game in which they tossed a ball with two others. When the others stopped sharing the ball with the subject, "the pain they felt at being cut out was devastating, on par with breaking a leg". "The conclusion [to the study]" wrote journalist and author Bruce Feiler, "[is that] while getting lots of likes or retweets feels great, the feeling of rejection from *not* getting them is often greater. People's fear of being excluded is intense."[15]

So, letting go of being liked is not about cutting off everyone who disagrees with you. It's more about being selective about whose connections and approval you value in the first place. As the saying goes, "You can't change the people around you, but you can change the people around you." Read that again!

If you're starting something new and feeling isolated, then joining communities, even if only online, can be extremely powerful. A quick Google or a search on social media will reveal communities in almost any area you can think of: female entrepreneurship, books, crafting, setting up an Etsy shop, film criticism, baking, freelancing... anything! Reach out to people online or in person, or join in with their events or groups. Try out a few, see what gels best for you, and be persistent.

It's amazing how open people can be to others who are in the same boat as them. While I don't agree with asking busy and experienced people if you can have coffee to "pick their brains" for free (if you want their expertise beyond asking one or two questions, you need to pay for it), the peer-to-peer support from online or real-life groups can be huge – especially if you have no-one in your immediate circle who understands what you're doing.

Because there *will* be struggles, no question. Even several years into my journey of "doing my own thing", I still have dark days of total self-doubt, wondering what on earth I'm doing. I still have days where every negative thing anyone has ever said about me comes back to haunt me and plays on a loop in my brain. And if you're anything like me, you will have those days too. It doesn't mean the critics are right. It just means you're human, which is where meditation can help.

The "shitty first draft"

Not to be dramatic, but with most new things in life, you're going to absolutely suck at them when you first start. (This can make other people's criticism even harder to bear, as we worry that maybe they're right.) I know this is a difficult pill to swallow for ambitious women like me and you. This is common. Dr Jessamy Hibberd, clinical psychologist and author of the book *The Imposter Cure*, calls this the Natural Genius tendency.[16] Just as it sounds, people who are like this generally find most things easy, and mainly enjoy doing things that come naturally to them. Many of us who identify as ambitious, anxious women will recognize this.

And there's nothing inherently wrong with that. It's nice to do what comes naturally to us, and it can be great – and sometimes necessary – to play to our strengths. But the problem with *only* doing this is that it can keep us small, stuck and boring. It limits us to what we're already good at, and stops us from trying new things just because we want to. It also keeps us caught in comparison, feeling that other people are naturally talented at stuff that we would love to be good at. We feel that because we're not naturally gifted at it, then there's no point in us even trying. This mindset keeps us stuck.

Don't get me wrong; it's totally understandable. People often go to great lengths to make their lives look effortless, and we all know the old "highlight reel" saying about people on social media: no-one is posting their failures. But thinking that everyone who's successful is just super-talented and has never had to work at anything, keeps us stuck and bitter, and limits our potential – and therefore, our whole life. There's a saying in the business world that you cannot publish your hilarious, perfect 200th podcast episode without first releasing the terrible, awkward AF first one. (I know this from personal experience!)

Author Anne Lamott calls this the "shitty first draft",[17] and another common phrase in business states: "If you're not embarrassed by the first thing you release/do/write, then you've waited too long to do it." This is about rewiring our entire mindset. Psychologist Dr Carol S. Dweck has written an entire book called, appropriately, *Mindset*,[18] to detail the exact mental reframe we're aiming for here. She calls it the "fixed mindset" versus the "growth mindset".

Long story short, in a "fixed mindset" we believe that our talents are stuck. We reason that we were born with them, or learned them early on, and there's not a lot we can do to change them. This means that when we find something tough, or we fail, we think that's the way it is. End of story. We might spend time and energy trying to prove to ourselves and everyone else how good we are at other stuff, to compensate for this. We believe that putting lots of effort in is futile and embarrassing, because we won't improve much anyway. We think success comes from talent, which we either have or don't. We believe everything should be effortless if we are good enough at it. We're stuck, we feel bad about it, and we're vulnerable to others' judgements as a result.

But in a "growth" mindset, we know success is about hard work, and not giving up; and that even talented people have to put in hours of practice to reach mastery. Rather than seeing hard work as something humiliating, we see it as proof of how committed we are.

This mindset isn't always spoken about. We love to hear about people's success, but we don't want to hear about the hours of work or struggle it took them to get there. We want to take a magic pill to fast forward through our problems, and we aren't happy when we're told that the practice *is* the solution. Just as with sitting down to meditate, the journey *is* the destination.

In popular culture, often, we like to skip the hard work. We like people who are light-hearted and say, "Oh, it was nothing!".

We reward modesty, especially in women. We expect them to break barriers, but we expect them to be a bit shambolic and slapdash too, as if working hard for something is shameful or nerdy or a bit too brash, and so women often apologize for their successes, as if it all sort of happened by accident or luck.

The growth mindset

Well, fuck that. With the growth mindset that meditation facilitates, we learn that working hard for something should be celebrated! Success feels much better when you know you have earned it, and – through your own grit and focus – overcame the judgements that may have been stacked against you.

When you know that success takes hard work (on top of any existing talent or privileges, which should not be discounted either), you can, paradoxically, face failure without being cowed by it, and in doing so, make success much more likely. You're golden.

(Attention: *This "hard work" idea is not an excuse to work yourself to burnout.* Persistence doesn't have to mean pain. See the next chapter for more on this.)

But to get to that success, you usually have to start small, and to be bad at it first. That's what meditation teaches us to do. Because no-one, in the history of the world, has ever been good at meditation on their first try. When it comes to trying new things, meditation is your friend. By its very practice, it helps us test this "fixed versus growth" mindset concept safely, without throwing ourselves into the deep end every time. It prepares us mentally for those times when we *do* need to throw ourselves into the depths and find out whether we can swim.

If we expect to be fabulous at something the first time we try it, we'll probably be stratospherically disappointed and give up when we're very much not. Artist Justine Hwang, who teaches calligraphy, says that she never expects anyone who is starting out to be good. On my podcast, she told me, "I always want my new students to feel safe to explore, and to fail, and to be bad at it. I spend a lot of time setting the ground rules. The perfection police are not allowed here. There's no fast-tracking it."[19]

After all, there's nothing more humbling than seeing those amazing videos of beautiful brush lettering on perfect milk-white parchment... and your own attempt looking like a sad scribble by Edward Scissorhands.

And it was Justine who first told me about this incredible quote, by Ira Glass, producer and host of NPR radio show, *This American Life*. It reads:

"Nobody tells this to people who are beginners; I wish someone had told me. All of us who do creative work, we get into it because we have good taste. But there is this gap. For the first couple of years you make stuff, it's just not that good.... It has potential, but it's not. But your taste – the thing that got you into the game – is still killer. And your taste is why your work disappoints you. A lot of people never get past this phase; they quit.

"Most people I know who do interesting, creative work went through years of this. We know our work doesn't

have this special thing. ... We all go through this. And if you are just starting out or you are still in this phase, you gotta know it's normal and the most important thing you can do is do a lot of work.

"It is only by going through a volume of work that you will close that gap, and your work will be as good as your ambitions. And I took longer to figure out how to do this than anyone I've ever met. It's gonna take a while. It's normal to take a while. You've just gotta fight your way through."[20]

In the meditation and mindfulness world, we have a phrase to describe this: "beginner's mind". It's the idea that when we sit down to meditate – to do anything – we need to approach it as a beginner – as if we've never done it before. We can never do the same meditation practice twice, even if we're listening to the exact same guided audio, because we're always different, and we notice new things every time. This approach encourages us to get curious, and makes us less likely to get totally distracted when we sit.

And, of course, the *point* of meditation isn't to be good at it.

And when we apply this to the rest of our lives, our inner critic loses her power. If we tell her that we don't expect things to be perfect in the first place, she's lost. The goal is to bring your negative inner critic along for the ride, and transform her into your biggest supporter. If the voice in your head is going to be there, she might as well help.

The point isn't to switch your inner voice off, or silence all criticism completely – it's to stop looking for evidence that you should quit, and give your inner voice evidence that you're on the right track, instead.

Remember: Hurt people hurt people

As well as rewiring our inner critic, becoming our own biggest supporter – no matter what anyone else thinks – makes working on our own sense of self centrally important. Mindfulness offers us some excellent tools to support us in this. It gives us an unparalleled chance to get familiar with what's inside our own heads; we can work through any resentment about other people's judgement without it overflowing or, worse, staying bottled up inside us and making us depressed.

We can really *feel* those feelings, accept them, *forgive ourselves* for all those less-than-comfortable thoughts, and let them go. We can get comfortable in our own skin, and build up our sense of purpose and resilience. We can also recognize that if someone is being rude or judgemental toward us, then it's probably because what we're doing or who we are is threatening them in some way. As that often-quoted phrase tells us, "Don't let people who didn't follow their dreams stop you from following yours." We can offer these people compassion; understand that if someone else feels trapped in their boring job or life, it must be galling to see you doing something different.

If you take time out of your day to meditate and strengthen your own compassion, you can begin to see yourself from another perspective – and in doing so, protect yourself from external judgement. You're taking back control of your own self-worth, and becoming far less vulnerable to what others say, think or do.

Of course, this doesn't make others' behaviour OK. Sometimes, we need to set tough boundaries for people who won't – or can't – be respectful. Working to become your own best supporter, helped by choice people in your life, can heal your heart when others break it by not being the supportive friends or family members you wanted them to be. Eventually, your heart becomes so strong and full that you feel OK, no matter what. At that point, you're basically bulletproof, and way happier.

MEDITATION TOOL

Visualization for self-possession

Once seated in meditation, close your eyes if you like. Notice your body, curiously and gently, and feel how it is to be here in your body today, now.

Visualize yourself walking or sitting at the top of a hiking path. Take the last few steps, feeling the ground under your feet or whatever physical sensations you can notice...and yes! You're at the top of the path; you've made it! Tune in to your senses. What can you see? What do you hear – the birds in the trees? What can you feel – a breeze on your skin? Can you smell the grass or the pine trees?

Straighten your spine and lift your chin, and imagine golden sunlight beaming down its warmth and light over each part of your body. You might even put your hands on your hips, in a power pose.

Breathe, as you notice the warmth, and the feeling of power... of being here, the boss of all you survey. Notice the tingling, the energy.

When you're ready, open your eyes without moving your body just yet.

How do you feel?

8

Mindful Productivity

(Or, How to Get Shit Done Without Burning Out)

"Measure your worth by your dedication to your path,
not by your 'successes' and 'failures'."

Elizabeth Gilbert, author

I happen to think the work-life balance concept is bollocks. Not because I believe that balancing work and life is impossible, or that we should aspire to be productive all the time. I just believe that pitching work and life as opposites is hugely unhelpful.

Firstly, it suggests that the two are mutually exclusive, and distinctly separate. Secondly, it suggests that work needs to take up 50% of the equation, and that the whole rest of our life should fit into the other 50%, if that.

It's no wonder we so often feel that our work equals our value, that we describe ourselves by our job titles, and feel devastated if our career isn't fulfilling. We're taught, through our very language, to feel as though work is equal, if not more important, to what makes us feel *alive*. Maybe I'm taking the whole work-life balance concept a bit too literally. But the phrase seems especially telling in a society obsessed with work and productivity. And anyone who's ever worked knows that the 50/50 thing is a myth anyway. It's way more likely to be 60/40, 70/30, or 80/20 – weighted toward work This isn't good for us.

In fact, a Mental Health Foundation survey of British adults found that one third of respondents felt unhappy or very unhappy about the amount of time they devote to work, and more than 40% of employees said they were neglecting other aspects of their life because of the amount of time they spent working. This, the foundation said, could increase their vulnerability to mental health problems.[1]

The same survey found that as a person's weekly hours increase, so do their feelings of unhappiness. It said that the more hours you spend at work, the more hours outside of work you are likely to spend thinking or worrying about it. Not a great recipe for work-life balance! Even worse, the survey found that many more women (42%) report unhappiness than men (29%) due to work.[2] Similarly, a 2020 survey by the US initiative Project: Time Off, found that 40% of US Millennials identified with the term "work martyr", and 48% even thought this nickname was "well-earned", i.e., a badge of honour![3]

It seems that surprisingly little has changed since psychologist Mike S. Bernick wrote in 1981, in the scientific journal *Political Psychology,* "Many people relate self-esteem to having a job. It is widely said that persons find identity and value through a job."[4]

Recognizing the need to rebalance

I realized the full extent of my tendency to attach my worth as a person to how many hours I worked when I spent November 2018 in Bali, supposedly "living my dreams". As a freelancer and solo business owner, I was working remotely while I was away, which was expected. I hadn't planned for the stay to be a "holiday", and it wasn't. Even so, I was staying at a yoga retreat centre right next door to the legendary Yoga Barn in Ubud. One balmy evening, as I was nursing a bright pink dragonfruit cocktail, it suddenly hit me – like a heavy gong at a sound bath – that in the past week, I had spent more hours doing yoga than I had sitting in front of my laptop doing work.

I wish I could tell you that I felt at peace right then, certain that I was "living my best life" and that all was well. But honestly? I didn't. I was immediately consumed by guilt, shame and blame. As a solopreneur, my small business is me, myself and I. If I don't show up, nothing happens. So when I realized that I'd spent more time doing yoga than working, my brain went into inner bitch overdrive. "This is why you're not as successful as other people", it taunted me. "You're lazy, you'll never succeed, you don't want it enough, other people would never do this."

I was pretty shocked at how quickly my usual patterns came to the surface, telling me that my value was only measured by how many hours I worked. I was so ashamed about what I felt doing more hours of yoga than work *said* about me and my success. Later, though, I realized, "*Hello?!* This is *why* I wanted to work for myself in the first place. This is the goal!" Nothing is perfect, but this was pretty close. When I'd had time to calm down, I realized that this was the entire point. *This* was the so-called work-life balance I had been striving for the whole time – the "permission" and the space to prioritize things that weren't work, and enjoy them without guilt.

I realized that work is only one part of life. When I was away, I'd also been meeting new people, trying new foods, shopping, sleeping, reading, swimming, walking, sunbathing, exploring, learning. Why should we spend more time hunched over our laptops than, well, doing *anything else* that makes life worth living? Yes, work makes money, which we need to survive, but *not working* helps our mental health, which is also essential. If we focus on one to the exclusion of the other, we end up poorer, financially or emotionally.

Re-assessing our priorities

So why are we so obsessed with the idea that work is somehow the most valuable and notable thing about us? The current working model has us exchange our time for money, so we value ourselves and our skills based on the income they might provide. Inevitably, as a result, we end up defining ourselves in that way. Anything else – such as spending hours doing yoga, or enjoying a non-lucrative hobby – makes you "a bit of a drifter", "unambitious", "not focused", or worse, "doomed to fail". (FYI, your immediate reaction, negative or positive, to my yoga story back there might tell you a lot about how you feel about the connection between work, money and worth.)

Of course, I realize how privileged I am that I can even contemplate this. I'm by no means rich, but even on the very rare occasions that I spend more time doing yoga than work, although my earnings do take a hit, I can still afford to eat and keep a roof over my head.

I fully acknowledge the privilege of that, and do not mean to dismiss it. But that doesn't mean that my original point doesn't stand. It just means that our system is broken. The fact that so many people *have to* work all hours of the day in order to make enough to survive – and don't have the financial privilege that I do to focus on something else – shows how obsolete and rigid our current working model, and how low our expectations around work, really are.

Because everyone deserves a life outside of work, and the pursuit of something other than money and rigid workplace goals. If we want to live a fulfilled and more mindful life, our goal must surely be to work smarter, not harder, and see our work as just one facet of everything we do that makes up our life. Our goal should be to work in a way that doesn't see us as little machines, exchanging time for money. The 9-to-5 (more like 8-to-7) paradigm is based on a totally outdated system. It does nothing for our mental health, stress levels and sense of self-worth.

Advocates for a universal basic income (UBI) – which would give a certain amount of money every month to each citizen, regardless of job or income – know this; and the idea of supplementing people's incomes so they can avoid the spectre of poverty and live a happier, more balanced life, isn't new. Sir Thomas More suggested it as far back as his 1516 book *Utopia*,[5] while Martin Luther King Jr proposed the idea of "guaranteed income" in his 1967 book *Where Do We Go from Here: Chaos or Community?*[6]

Basic Income UK, which is a member of the Unconditional Basic Income Europe (UBI-Europe) alliance, says that UBI would help us "to rethink how and why we work, contribute to better working conditions, reduce inequality and extreme financial poverty, and contribute to fewer working hours and better distribution of jobs".[7] Sounds good to me.

As I write this, the world is still navigating the impact of the COVID-19 pandemic on remote working, and what the long-term effects may be. In my view, this shift away from office presenteeism and living our lives in the office can't come soon enough.

I have a vivid memory from when I was still working in a 9-to-5 job, with a three-hour commute. I was hanging up wet clothes at half past midnight after an evening of shopping, cooking dinner, life admin and washing, and had my alarm set for 6:30am so that I could do it all again the next day. I wondered who the actual *hell* had designed modern life so that work took up the vast majority of it, and everything else had to be squished into a handful of hours on either side. It's totally nonsensical, and does a disservice to who we all are as varied, creative, sensitive, interesting, mindful humans. When so many of us can now work from anywhere, at any time, no matter what the time zone, as long as we have a laptop and an internet connection, why does the time-for-money, 9-to-5 (usually longer), eight-hours-a-day, five-days-a-week, one-chair-in-one-physical-office structure still hold so much sway?

I acknowledge that not everyone can, or even wants to, work from home or redesign their entire day flexibly. In fact, one recent article by Professor Jan-Emmanuel De Neve, director of Oxford University's Wellbeing Research Centre, said that:

"Building meaningful relationships with co-workers… is critical to job and life satisfaction. Working from home all the time simply does not allow for that to the same extent as the office.

"And work itself represents much more than a pay cheque – it is essential to one's social identity. We know from prior research that when somebody loses their job, half of the negative impact on wellbeing stems not from the loss of income, but from the loss of social ties, identity, and a routine that comes with a job."[8]

But for many of us (and I would argue, most of us, as human beings), flexible and mindful working – and a life that doesn't entirely revolve around work – is a major positive. And, sorry, Professor De Neve, but if commuting to and from an office is "essential to our social identity", then I'd gently suggest we may want to consider why that is and change *that*, rather than cling on to an office job that's otherwise making us ill with misery.

Burnout blues

And this goes beyond my simple hatred of the daily commute. Studies show that when work becomes all-consuming and squeezes out everything else that makes life worth living, the consequences can be dire. The 2020 Labour Force Survey (LFS) in the UK found that 17.9 million working days were lost in 2019–2020 due to work-related stress, depression and anxiety, and that "the rate of self-reported work-related stress, depression or anxiety has increased in recent years." The survey also found that women "have statistically significantly higher rates" of this, especially "in age groups 25 to 34, and 35 to 44", with the main causes reported as "workload, tight deadlines, too much work, too much pressure."[9]

Such issues can lead to burnout, and are a leading cause of chronic stress, which can lead to all sorts of major health and social problems long-term, as well as making us utterly miserable. Ironically, it also makes us less productive and far less good at our jobs, too. Famously, in 2019, the World Health Organization said that burnout is an actual syndrome resulting from "chronic workplace stress that has not been successfully managed". It said that it is characterised by "feelings of energy depletion or exhaustion", "increased mental distance from one's job, or feelings of negativism or cynicism related to one's job", and "a sense of ineffectiveness and lack of accomplishment", and recognized it as an occupational phenomenon.[10] To which, my super-professional response would be, "About bloody time."

According to non-profit Mayo Foundation for Medical Education and Research, "burnout" includes the following symptoms.[11]

How many do you recognize?

BURNOUT QUIZ

Answer yes/no and count up the number of yes answers.
1. Becoming cynical or critical at work. Y/N
2. Dragging yourself to work and having trouble getting started. Y/N

---

3. Becoming irritable or impatient with co-workers, customers or clients. Y/N
4. Lacking the energy to be consistently productive. Y/N
5. Finding it hard to concentrate. Y/N
6. Lacking satisfaction from your achievements. Y/N
7. Feeling disillusioned about your job. Y/N
8. Using food, drugs or alcohol to feel better, or to numb your feelings. Y/N
9. A change in sleep habits. Y/N

How many did you get?
1–3: Slight spark
4–6: Fighting flames
7–9: Burned to a crisp

When I worked in an office, I'd have said "yes" to every single thing on that list. And if you can relate to this, you're not alone.

A survey of 7,500 full-time employees by US polling agency Gallup found that 23% said they felt burned out more often than not, and an additional 44% said they felt burned out sometimes.[12] This means that nearly two-thirds of full-time workers are dealing with burnout at any given point!

However, some forward-thinking companies *are* starting to realize that more work, more hours, and rigid presenteeism does not necessarily equal better work or mental health. The idea of a four-day working week, for example, is gathering support. In the UK in 2018, the Trades Union Congress (TUC) found that "8 in

10 workers (81%) want to reduce working time in the future – with 45% opting for a four-day working week." They advised that "The UK should consider how to move to a four-day week over the course of this century."[13]

Andrew Barnes, author of the book *The 4 Day Week* (not to be confused with *The 4-Hour Work Week* by Tim Ferriss,[14] which takes the idea even further!), has said, "The reality is that... you are only productive approximately three hours a day. So, the problem is that we use time as a surrogate for understanding productivity seriously."[15] Anyone who's sat at work counting down the minutes until they are "allowed" to leave, or seething with rage at how they have to ask their boss "permission" to take time off or do something other than work, will feel this acutely.

In fact, in a famous 2019 trial, Microsoft found that when it gave staff Fridays off, there was a 40% rise in productivity.[16] And in 2020, a group of cross-party MPs – including Green Party MP Caroline Lucas – wrote an open letter to the *Independent* newspaper saying that:

"A four-day week would bring multiple benefits to society, the environment, our democracy, and our economy (through increased productivity)." It added, "One of the biggest impacts would be better mental health and wellbeing across the board, with more time available for socializing, family and community.

"... Three quarters of UK workers already supported a four-day working week before the coronavirus pandemic hit and millions of workers have now had a taste of working remotely and on different hours. It's in no one's interests

to return back to the pressure and stress that people were under before this pandemic."[17]

Maybe by the time this book comes out, changing technology and the impact of the Covid-19 pandemic will mean that companies that used to have a zero-tolerance policy for flexible working or for working from home might have come to their senses, and realized that allowing employees to fit their work around their life, rather than the other way round, is the only sane policy. In the meantime, it is unfortunately (or fortunately, depending on how you look at it) up to us to make work... *work* for us, and not the other way round.

Make mindful productivity your new goal

If you want to be happier at work, to find your own sweet spot of "getting shit done" without burning out, and have time to do other stuff you enjoy, to rest *and* spend time with your partner or family too, then the real question is not: "How can I get a better work-life balance?", but: "How can I fit work in around my life, and not the other way around?" This is what I call *mindful productivity*. It means seeing rest, play, creativity, your social life, and your hobbies as *just* as important, if not more so, than work. Because you can't meditate burnout away without fixing the root cause.

In his book *Company of One*, Paul Jarvis relates the story of Miranda Hixon, a designer, who intentionally keeps her business small, so she can make what she needs, without constantly striving for more. Jarvis writes:

"Miranda has found a way to have enough responsibility to succeed on her own terms, but not so much responsibility that she becomes stressed... Able to retreat for long stretches of time to a yurt she built in the Sierra Nevada foothills, she finds that her overall life is less stressed, as well."[18]

Even if we can't all escape to a yurt in the mountains just yet (I'm working on it!), we can still learn from Miranda's story. Honour rest. Plan life and work around it, rather than seeing it as what we do when work is done. (Let's be honest; that basically never happens!) This can help us to get *more* accomplished in the long-run. Paradoxically, mindful productivity enables us to *achieve more,* by *doing less.*

But how? Three words: Meditation. Builds. Focus. Focus on why, what, and how we're doing. Fewer distractions. Less time spent on "busy work" that doesn't move the needle on our goals. Less patience for work that we hate; accepting poor pay for too-long hours; or sitting there for our allotted eight hours a day, because that's what we've always done.

Once we realize that work is not about how much time we spend on something, but the tasks we accomplish – whether it takes us ten minutes or ten hours – we are free. And this concept only becomes more relevant, the more experienced we get. As the much-shared, brilliant quote goes: "If I do a job in 30 minutes, it's because I spent 10 years learning how to do it in 30 minutes. You owe me for the years, not the minutes." How amazing would it be if we could actually *reduce* our workday, the more experienced we became?

And, to get stuff done efficiently in an ever-busier, distracted, time-poor world, we need to train our *attention*. We need to know how to focus. At its most basic, meditation is attention training. It's about choosing a goal, staying laser-focused on it, and getting it done – without overthinking, reaching burnout, procrastinating or experiencing overwhelming anxiety.

Finding focus

Psychologist, long-time meditator and author of *Focus*, Daniel Goleman, describes "inner focus" as "the driver of excellence", and calls it "self-awareness and self-management".[19] In an interview with *Forbes* magazine, he said:

> *"[It's] how well we can tune in to our guiding values... and handle distressing emotions so they don't interfere with getting things done, marshal positive emotions to stay motivated... and bounce back from setbacks."*[20]

It's clear that getting focused is a good thing, especially if you have big ambitions. In fact, psychologists generally agree that there are five types of attention. For Goleman and Davidson, whose amazing book, *The Science of* Meditation, I've already referred to in this book, these types are listed as:

- Selective attention: the capacity to focus on one element and ignore others.

- Vigilance: maintaining a constant level of attention as time goes by.
- Allocating: noticing small or rapid shifts in what we experience.
- Goal focus: or "cognitive control" – keeping a specific goal or task in mind despite distractions.
- Meta-awareness: being able to track the quality of your awareness – for example, noticing your mind wandering or when you've made a mistake.[21]

When it comes to getting things done, we all use all the types, but selective attention is arguably the most important one to master. Luckily, meditation helps.

As Goleman and Davidson explain, a study by Amishi Jha, an associate psychology professor, and her team at the University of Miami, found that beginners who trained in Mindfulness-Based Stress-Reduction (MBSR) – the standard eight-week mindfulness course by pioneer Dr Jon Kabat-Zinn in the US – significantly improved their selective attention.[22]

Because meditation strengthens our prefrontal cortex and dampens down our amygdala, it allows us to focus deliberately on a specific thing, rather than being distracted by a passing thought or emotion (or an Instagram feed). It might also be considered as what psychologist Mihaly Csikszentmihalyi calls "flow" in his classic book, *Flow: The Psychology of Happiness.* In his words:

"Attention is like energy in that without it, no work can be done... One needs to learn to control attention... [through] meditation and prayer if one is so inclined. ...

The important thing is to enjoy the activity for its own sake, and to know that what matters is not the result, but the control one is acquiring over one's attention."[23]

Remember how I said earlier that becoming the world's best meditator isn't the goal? At its most basic level, improving our attention stops our mind from getting lost and distracted, which is usually a good thing when it comes to feeling happier.

Daydreaming can be glorious – we've all had great ideas in the shower! – but studies pioneered by Marcus Raichle, a neuroscientist at Washington University in St Louis, US, show that when we're not focusing on much, our brains are "noisier" than when we're working on something engaging. The studies showed that these wandering thoughts usually drift toward the negative, to ourselves, and how we're doing (or, more likely, *not* doing). Raichle's research found that when we'reostensibly doing nothing, the part of our brains known as the midline prefrontal cortex (mPFC) and the post-cingulate cortex (the PCC) connect together and "chat", making our mind pretty active even when we're supposedly "at rest".

This means that when left to our own devices – or what Raichle called the brain's "default mode", – rather than getting lost in lovely daydreaming, we actually tend to spiral into unhelpful, ruminating, damaging or anxiety-inducing thoughts – especially if we're feeling stressed.[24]

This effect has been further confirmed recent studies by addiction specialists, psychiatrists and neuroscientists Dr Judson Brewer and Kathleen Garrison, and their teams at Yale and Brown University.[25] Another study at Harvard University even led researchers to conclude that "A wandering mind is an unhappy mind."[26]

Training our attention through meditation allows us to notice when this is happening, so that we can bring ourselves back to the present, improve our focus, get more done in less time, and stay a whole lot happier as a result. Mindfulness-based techniques and principles can help in a practical, tangible way, too.

Here are some of my favourite ways to get and stay more focused. I have tried all of them, and I recommend them to my clients. Remember though, these are only suggestions. As usual, working mindfully is about finding out what works for you.

Meditative brain dump

Begin your workday with a short, focused attention meditation. Do a body scan, and check in with how you're feeling. Come back to your breath when you get distracted. Once you're feeling grounded and alert, allow your mind to run through your to-do list or priorities. Ask yourself a question if you need to. Allow whatever comes to mind to appear. Afterwards, jot down whatever came up, while you remember it, if it helps. This can help clear your mind and get your worries or priorities down on paper so they're not swirling around in your head.

A short to-do list

Even if you have umpteen thousand things on your brain dump list, keep your actual daily "to-do" list very, very short. Aim to get between one or two – or at a push, three! – major things done per day, and consider anything else a bonus.

Day blocking

Remember at school when you had Art on Tuesday, and double Maths on Thursday (urgh)? Day blocking is like that, but for adult life. Set specific days to do certain things, such as "podcast editing" on Tuesday, "writing" on Wednesday, or "client calls" on Thursday. This helps you stay focused, without constantly hopping from task to task.

Batching

Take "day blocking" a step further by batching tasks. For example, on the first Monday of the month, rather than planning your social media posts for the next week, you could spend a bit longer planning them for the entire month. That way, next Monday, you'll have freed up time for something else. This doesn't work for everyone – I often like to be a bit more spontaneous and only plan a week or two in advance – but some people swear by it, and I can see why.

Time/hour blocking

Some like to plan their day in blocks of hours, to get more done, more efficiently. For example, they might have a "morning routine" block from 7–8am, an "admin" block from 8–10am, and a "work" block from 2–4pm. That way, they share out their time and don't feel guilty if they're not working all the time. It also takes the willpower out of it – you just do the thing when it's time, rather than agonizing over whether you *feel like* doing it.

The Pomodoro® Technique

This is a time management method developed by consultant Francesco Cirillo in the late 1980s.[27] It takes its name from the classic "tomato" timer (*pomodoro* means *tomato* in Italian). You set a timer for 25 minutes, work, and when it goes off, make a note of it. Then take a five-minute break. After four intervals, take a 15–20-minute break before starting again. There are hundreds of apps that can do this for you, but I just use my phone and a Post-It note!

Just five minutes

When a task is so challenging or boring that you can't even bear the thought of doing it for 25 minutes – such as a jog in the rain, maybe, or filing your tax return – tell yourself you'll start with five minutes. Getting started is often the hardest part, and after that, you can usually go for longer. Even if you intend to literally do five minutes, challenge yourself to see how much you can get done in that time. Usually, it's enough to motivate you to do a bit more.

Habit/task tracking + rewards

I have an entire "how to" for this in Chapter 4, but, long story short, tracking involves setting a specific goal, and then tracking when you do it. That way, you can see at a glance how you're doing, and assign yourself a reward when you achieve your goal. Psychology shows that working toward pleasurable rewards, and ticking off a habit each time you do it, helps you count the small wins along the way, and build up a consistent habit that helps toward your long-term goal.

Building non-work, pleasurable things into the day

Talking of rewards, I find that building nice things into your day helps overall productivity, so the workday doesn't feel like one long slog. This is way easier to do if you work from home and don't have back-to-back meetings, obviously. But if you can, I suggest building in "non-work" things at intervals – and not just social media scrolling! This could be ten minutes of reading a book, lighting a candle or using your favourite hand cream and stopping to breathe in the scent. It helps you take back control of your time without being too disruptive, and reminds you that you are not only your work.

Workday movement, e.g., yoga, dancing or a walk

Similarly, they say that "A change is as good as a rest." This can definitely be true when it comes to work. Taking a few minutes between tasks can energize our working day routine, even if we don't have time for a full break. You could do some stretches, a quick walk, or play your favourite song and have a little dance. When you get back to work, you'll definitely feel better than if you'd stayed sitting and scrolling.

Writing a "to-done" list and closing down the day

For such a simple idea, this can be life-changing! Rather than lamenting what you didn't get done at the end of the day, instead, write a quick list of what you *did* get done. Everything counts. It's so easy to lie in bed at night tormenting ourselves with what we didn't achieve, and forget to give ourselves credit for what we *did* do. This "to-done" list helps put our minds at rest, and reminds us not to always be chasing the next thing. I'm usually surprised at how much I got done, even on a day where I felt as useless as pineapple on pizza.

Beyond focus: your human needs

Working mindfully isn't just about honing your attention to within an inch of its life, or keeping your to-do list short. It's also about being mindful about *why* you're doing something, and managing your time in a way that supports your mental health and leisure goals.

Your why

We can't get fully mindfully productive until we address where we're going in the first place – and why. That's why vision boards are so popular. Visualizing where we're going, and knowing why we're doing something, will always keep us going far more effectively than doing something without knowing the reason for it.

The analogy about the plane flying from New York City to Tokyo – or the "one degree effect" – explains this perfectly. The rules of air navigation state that for every degree a plane veers off its course, it misses its target destination by one mile for every 60 miles it flies. That means that if a plane takes off in NYC but stays one degree off course for the entire 6,700 miles, it will end up 112 miles away from Tokyo, hovering somewhere above the Pacific Ocean instead of arriving at its destination. Not ideal.

We can think of having an end goal – a compelling "why" – in a similar way. Of course, there's only so much we can control in life, and sometimes we set our final destination with no idea how we're going to get there. Maybe our dreams are so massive that we don't yet know how we can make them a reality. And just because we've flown off course at some point, doesn't mean we can't course-correct along the route.

But that doesn't mean we shouldn't set a goal or destination in the first place. As Nicole Antoinette, creator of the Real Talk Radio podcast, says, "You learn how to do the thing by doing the thing... You don't have to be strong enough on day one to get to year ten."[28]

That's why I always ask my clients to start with their "why".

- Why do you want to do what you're doing?
- What's your end goal?
- How do you want to feel when you arrive at "success"?
- What does success look and feel like for you?
- Who do you need to be to get there?
- What is your main motivation for change?
- What is most important to you overall?
- What needs to change in your life and mindset right now to be that person?
- Why are you working so hard on this thing in the first place?

My guess is that your goal it isn't to "burn out completely, damage your mental and physical health, and never have time to rest or make a dent in your massive 'to-read' pile of fiction books".

(Sidenote: the Japanese have a word for your "to-read" list, which is "tsundoku" (積ん読). It translates as "Gathering reading materials but letting them pile up in one's home without reading them", and is "also used to refer to books ready for reading later when they are on a bookshelf". Isn't that brilliant?!)[29]

Mindful productivity, and truly balancing work with life in a way that makes sense for you, is about understanding your core values, and defining what success means to you... whether that's travelling the world First Class, or having time to sit outside with the sun on your face, a coffee in hand and a dog at your feet.

A great exercise for this comes from the leadership coach, Tony Robbins. I definitely don't agree with everything he says or does, but me and my clients use this particular concept to great effect.

THE SIX CORE HUMAN NEEDS

This is based on the idea that humans need six things to feel good and purposeful. To figure out how you feel about your situation now, versus your "dream life", or end goal, ask yourself:

1. Certainty: How does your situation bring certainty to your life (or not)?
2. Variety: How does your life meet, or not meet, your need for variety?
3. Significance: How does your life make you feel significant in your field?
4. Love and connection: Where does your sense of love and connection come from?
5. Growth: Where are you growing, or not? Are there more opportunities for this?

6. Contribution: How are you contributing, or not? How would you like to?

When we really struggle to make changes – especially in our work – it can be because we're afraid of losing one of these core needs, even if, on the surface, the new career or skill is absolutely something we want. To figure this out for yourself, I recommend asking yourself the above questions, and journaling on how your current lifestyle, working day, or career satisfies each need in turn, even if it seems counterintuitive. Then, do the same exercise for your "dream" or ideal life or career.

For each need, identify how your current, or "old", life, satisfies it. Then, journal on how your future life will look, for each. Dream big, here. For example, you may be dreaming of leaving your 9-to-5 job, but the core need of Certainty is so important to you that the idea of leaving a regular wage behind is terrifying. Or maybe you hate your actual day-to-day job, but you love the Connection you have with your colleagues and industry peers.

Perhaps in your ideal life, you'd sacrifice Certainty by leaving behind a regular wage, but you'd gain hugely in Variety, by choosing a new career that is far more varied and interesting than your old one. Maybe you'd lose Connection with your current colleagues, but rediscover it with new clients? It's up to you. At the end of the exercise, you'll have a much clearer idea of what's important to you, what might be holding you back, and what's driving you to change or keep going.

The value of values

Working through these core needs can also help you to dig deep into what your true values and priorities are. When all is said and done:

- What's important to you?
- What would you love your best friends to say about you when you're not in the room?
- What would you want to be remembered for?

Will you be remembered like "She was a reliable and loyal friend", or, "She enjoyed her life and followed her curiosity", or "She spent hours scrolling news online, and always stayed in the office for hours after her boss left"? That may seem a bit morbid, but Buddhists spend a heck of a lot of time contemplating their own death as a way to sharpen their focus on what's truly important in life, so if it's good enough for them, it's good enough for me. There's even a "mindfulness" phone app called WeCroak, which does nothing except alert you: "Don't forget, you're going to die!" at random intervals throughout the day, for this exact reason. The app description reads: "Find happiness by contemplating your mortality... Each day, we'll send you five invitations at randomized times to stop and think about death. It's based on a Bhutanese folk saying that to be a happy person one must contemplate death five times daily. The WeCroak invitations come at random times and at any moment. Just like death."[30]

Even if that's a bit too dark for you right now, I personally find it becomes a lot easier to figure out why you're working so hard and making such big changes in your life when you get a little perspective, decide what your values are, and muster the courage to follow them. Of course, sometimes you have to work late, or an unavoidable commitment or unmissable opportunity comes up. It happens. But one of my main motivations for setting up my own business was to ensure that I had more quality time with my partner, and reminding myself of that helps guide my decisions and ethos, so I prioritize spending time with him over late meetings. (And I once had a job interview that I asked to rearrange because my then-partner had been rushed into hospital, and the negative reaction I had from the interviewer about it made me glad I'd dodged that bullet. I cancelled the interview completely.)

For you, it might be different. You might not have this luxury right now; you might have to work night shifts, or do evening meetings, or miss dinner. But prioritizing your values can still be the end goal. I worked for years before I was able to make that change, and I still work at it. But at least when you know what your values are, you know what you're aiming for – your end destination.

When I was a staff journalist, I dreamed of getting the word "editor" in my job title. And when I finally did, even though I was desperate to leave and didn't really care about the job anymore, I still worried about letting the certainty of that title go. After I left, I struggled with what to call myself when people asked what I do. Turns out that the title gave me more certainty and significance than I had realized.

In the end though, by reminding myself of my values, I realized that my job *title* didn't matter half as much as doing something I enjoyed; and working to build a business that was mine, rather than working for somebody else. I now seek significance in other ways – doing something I believe in, putting content out there that I feel proud of, being a good friend and partner, prioritizing my health and rest, learning new skills... It's definitely not always easy to adjust your values and practise what you preach, but it makes decisions in your life and work a heck of a lot easier when you know what's really important to you.

Becoming mindfully productive and successful isn't about living up to other people's values or doing what other people find impressive. Being mindfully productive is the equivalent of setting your destination, defiantly, as Tokyo or Paris or Sydney, and knowing that even if you get a bit lost on the way, or you don't know anyone else who's been there, you have faith that you'll course-correct as you fly.

You are not your work

Finding this sort of "mindful success" and work balance means building up a solid sense of who you are. It means knowing yourself so well that you not only know your values and core needs, but you have the courage to stand by those convictions when they're challenged, too.

Luckily, meditation provides tools to help us do just that.

Not only does the practice help us – as I always say – to get to know ourselves, but Buddhism also offers us a nice little framework for how to apply the practice to our lives. This is known as the Noble Eightfold Path. It is not intended to be followed in order; more used as a general guideline for life.

To summarize very simply, it is:

- Right understanding: understanding how things are, and that your actions have consequences.
- Right thought: working to build a loving, non-selfish and non-violent state of mind.
- Right speech: speaking truthfully and not in a malicious way that harms others.
- Right action: behaving in a moral, peaceful and honourable way. Showing integrity.
- Right livelihood: not making a living in a way that harms others.
- Right effort: the desire to cultivate a good, wholesome state of mind.
- Right mindfulness: to be aware of your mind, body, thoughts, feelings and ideas.
- Right concentration: working to set aside worry or doubt, and instead cultivate a happier, more peaceful mind.[31]

These points ask us to check in with ourselves and course-correct on our plane journey.

Similarly, on a more secular level, Mindfulness-based Cognitive Therapy (MBCT) is careful to make sure all of its students learn the Seven Principles of Mindfulness. These "seven pillars" are also known as "the seven attitudes", as laid out by the mindfulness specialist Jon Kabat-Zinn.

They are:

- Non-judging: awareness, and not judging things as black or white, good or bad.

- Patience: understanding that things happen in good time; there's no need to rush ahead.
- Beginner's mind: life is always changing; you can never know or control everything.
- Trust: knowing yourself, being open to others but ultimately trusting your own mind.
- Non-striving: recognizing that you are enough in the present moment.
- Acceptance: not resignation, but a clear-eyed view of how things are right now.
- Letting go: working to be free from worry, and being present in the here and now.[32]

I find "Non-striving" to be the most relevant to our work here. It means that we are enough, and we don't always have to be striving to do or be more all the time. Through this lens, even more important than work-life balance is "work-self-worth" balance – the idea that we are not our work, and that we should not value ourselves by our productivity and achievements.

Achievement and getting great stuff done can be awesome, but it's not everything we are, or are not. As the saying goes: "*Your worth is not determined by your productivity.*" When it comes to figuring out a more mindful approach toward work, it can be helpful to remember that our worth as a human, our values and how we spend our time cannot be measured by our output, the number of hours spent staring at a screen, or the number of zeroes at the end of our bank balance.

All humans need a mix of achievement and rest, and I'm not arguing for one over the other. Having goals and ambition is a healthy part of life. But the choice shouldn't be "work hard, be productive and risk burnout", or "chill out, abandon your goals, and never achieve anything". We need both things to be happy, healthy humans. Sometimes, we maybe *do* want to work late or accept an opportunity that takes us away from our family or usual goals. And that's OK. The mindful part is in being aware of that – in realizing that life and work can balance in a way that is good for our wellbeing.

Meditation is often seen as a "helpful hack" to get us to optimize our attention and improve our focus, but this does it a disservice. We mustn't aim for focus at the expense of ethics or our own health.

Being truly mindfully productive isn't about purely "optimizing productivity" and "hacking our way" to someone else's idea of success. It's about finding our own definition, balancing our work with our values, and remembering that we are humans, not robots or corporate cogs in a big machine. It's about taking control of our own plane, and flying it wherever we want to – with less stress, less burnout, and more enjoyment, too. Win, win.

MEDITATION TOOL

Visualizations for focus

The waterfall

Once seated in meditation, imagine yourself sitting behind a big waterfall. You're safe and dry on a bit of rock, with the water rushing down in front of you. Whenever a distraction arises, allow the thought or stressful feeling to disappear down into the waterfall. Repeat.

The river

Once seated in meditation, imagine yourself sitting next to a flowing river, or on a rock in the middle of it. Whenever a distraction comes up, notice it, and imagine it floating away, gently, down the river. Bring your attention back to your body, solid and secure. Repeat.

The sky

Once seated in meditation, imagine yourself sitting under a clear blue sky. Your thoughts and distractions are clouds. Allow them to float past; let them go, and continue bringing your focus back to the wider blue sky behind the clouds. Repeat.

The Post-It note

Once seated in meditation, bring your focus to your breath, wherever you feel it most, especially in your nose, or between your eyes. Breathe normally. Whenever a thought arises, notice it, and imagine pinning the thought on a pinboard, or making a mark on a Post-It note, and sticking it just out of sight. Bring your focus back to your breath. Repeat.

The intentions

A great journaling exercise for this is to begin your day by jotting down some "intentions", answering questions such as, "What do I need today?", "What would bring me joy and strength today?", "What would be an ideal day for me today?" This can help focus your mind and go beyond a simple to-do list, to remind you of what's really important.

9

Meditation for Sleep

(or, Permanently Exhausted Pigeons)

"Sleep is the very best thing we can do for our brains. It's the way we love our minds. Sleep is basically self-respect."

Brené Brown, research professor and expert in vulnerability, shame and empathy

It may seem odd that this book has a chapter about sleep, given the rest of it is about being more aware and in Buddhist terms, meditation is about "waking up" to reality. But it's a fact that many people first come to meditation to find relaxation and sleep better. When I first started teaching meditation to busy, stressed and anxious women, I was surprised to find myself talking about sleep much more than I expected to.

The women I speak to want to be more alert, more aware, more energized. They want to love themselves more and have the courage and clarity to shine at work and in life. They want to take on the world. Never have they said, "Actually, I want to feel sleepy." But invariably, so many of us struggle with sleep, which actually makes it less likely that we'll ever feel like the badasses we want to be.

Any of these familiar to you?

YOUR RELATIONSHIP WITH SLEEP QUIZ

Answer yes/no and count up the number of yes answers.

1. Not sleeping enough. Y/N
2. Checking email and social media in bed. Y/N
3. Going to bed too late. Y/N
4. Not prioritizing sleep over work or Netflix. Y/N
5. Assuming getting five to six hours of sleep is enough. Y/N
6. "Saving up" lie-ins for the weekend. Y/N
7. Not allowing yourself time to wind down before bed. Y/N
8. Drinking caffeine after 2pm. Y/N
9. Drinking alcohol to make you drowsy. Y/N
10. Waking up in the night and not being able to go back to sleep. Y/N
11. Overthinking and a racing mind, even when in bed. Y/N
12. Getting up at night to do that "one thing" that's on your mind. Y/N
13. Feeling guilty about lie-ins or spending time sleeping. Y/N
14. Feeling guilty about wanting to rest. Y/N
15. Criticizing yourself for feeling tired. Y/N

16. Seeing the ability to "survive" on five hours' kip as a good thing, in yourself or others. Y/N

17. Thinking getting eight to nine hours' sleep a night is only for the lazy/lucky/deadly boring. Y/N

18. Secretly thinking the ability to sleep less is the secret to success. Y/N

19. Finding yourself in bed, trying to sleep, replaying that memory of being bullied in the playground aged ten, or *that* awkward conversation with your boss, over and over. Y/N

How many did you get?

1–5: Slightly stirring

6–12: One eye open

13–16: Tossing and turning

17–19: Utterly exhausted

If these sound like you, you're not alone. For so many of us, our relationship with sleep is broken. UK health agency Public Health England (PHE) joined forces with The Sleep Council to create a "Sleep and Recovery tooklit", after their research found that lost sleep costs the UK economy more than £30bn per year.[1]

Figures from the UK Office for National Statistics found that 67% of UK adults struggle with disrupted sleep, and almost a quarter (23%) get no more than five hours a night. Even more (26%) say that "improving sleep" is their biggest health ambition, but more than half (51%) don't take any measures to help them do that. And the same study found that on average, women get less sleep than men, at six hours per night rather than seven.[2]

In the US, the Sleep Foundation found that 35.2% of all adults reported sleeping on average fewer than seven hours a night, and that insufficient sleep had an economic impact of over $411bn each year in the US alone.[3]

"I'll sleep when I'm dead"

It's little wonder we're all so sleep deprived. There are so many bullshit ideas about sleep in our modern world – especially if we're ambitious, and always feel we should be doing more.

How many of these have you come across before?

- Millionaire entrepreneurs boasting about getting up at 4:30am (casually forgetting to mention this means they're tucked up in bed by 8pm).
- Thinking that extroverts who prioritize "fun" instead of sleep are more interesting than people who like to be tucked up on time.
- Attaching glamour and awe to jobs that require employees to work all night.
- Idolizing people who say they "manage" on five hours of sleep or get up at 5am.
- Seeing people who get up for dawn yoga as somehow better than the rest of us.

- Seeing people who are always busy and sleep less as more efficient, harder working, or somehow more deserving of success and happiness than others.
- Thinking that the only way to achieve real success is to sacrifice sleep.
- Thinking that you can catch up on sleep and rest when you're older.

When people tell me that their job requires them to stay at work until gone 11pm and then race back into the office the next morning, rather than being impressed by their commitment, I nod politely, privately thinking that they must be ragingly inefficient at their jobs, or – more likely – that their workplace is toxic, and/or terrible at managing staff workload.

In English, we even have phrases such as: "Sleep is for the weak", and "I'll sleep when I'm dead", just to ram the point home.

Well, I say "Hell no!" to all of that – and I encourage you to do the same. Getting enough sleep and prioritizing rest is crucial to our brain functioning, and our ability to feel happy and healthy in our bodies – both in the short-term, and for our long-term health as we age. Recent scientific research into the importance of sleep is unequivocal. It *proves* that the less you sleep, the more likely you are to be speeding toward an early grave, and to feel like crap as you do it.

PHE says that adults who sleep for fewer than six hours a night have a 13% higher mortality risk than adults who sleep for at least seven hours.[4] The excellent neuroscientist and sleep expert Matthew Walker summarizes, "The shorter your sleep, the shorter your life." In fact, Walker's bestselling book *Why We Sleep* explains in minute detail how and why getting eight to nine hours of sleep per night is non-negotiable, especially if you want to improve your physical and mental health. As Walker says:

> "When you are not getting enough sleep, you work less productively and thus need to work longer to accomplish a goal. This means you often must work longer and later into the evening, arrive home later, go to bed later, and need to wake up earlier, creating a negative feedback loop.
>
> "Why try to boil a pot of water on medium heat when you could do so in half the time on high? People often tell me that they do not have enough time to sleep because they have so much work to do.
>
> "Without wanting to be combative in any way whatsoever, I respond by informing them that perhaps the reason they still have so much to do at the end of the day is precisely because they do not get enough sleep at night."[5]

And, if that wasn't enough, he also drops this:

> "The leading causes of disease and death in developed nations – such as heart disease, [extreme] obesity, dementia, diabetes, and cancer – all have recognized causal links to a lack of sleep."[6]

A permanently exhausted pigeon

After I read Walker's book, I felt validated. Suddenly, if felt OK to prioritize sleep. Wanting more sleep is allowed! Encouraged! *Necessary*, even! Here was proof that we don't have to survive on five hours of sleep to prove to everyone that we are working hard enough to exist! We don't *have* to be exhausted all the time, trying to be superwoman, forcing ourselves to be ever more productive while sacrificing our health and sanity in the process. Turns out, it's just not true that we can live happily and productively on less sleep than we need. It's slowly killing us, and making us feel like shit.

As someone who's always loved my sleep and always felt like I needed more of it, this is welcome news. As a night owl in an early bird world, I'd always felt like a square peg trying to fit into a round hole, forcing myself out of bed to get an early train, stuck in a zombie trance until at least midday. The modern world is designed almost exclusively for early birds – with early rising so celebrated – forcing the entire world to fit into some archaic Industrial Revolution framework that just doesn't work for everyone.

I was chronically tired for most of my adult life, surviving on about six hours of sleep each night for ten years, wondering why I felt utterly terrible all the time. For years, I felt like there was something seriously wrong with me, and that I just needed to "get my shit together". It didn't occur to me that some of us might just have different "peak hours" to others. It was only when I started working for myself that I realized: "Oh, *this* is what getting enough sleep feels like!" It was genuinely life-changing. Suddenly, I had energy, and could actually think straight.

But whether you're a night owl or an early bird – or, as that popular meme would say, "a permanently exhausted pigeon" – one of the secrets to good sleep is finding out what works for you, and prioritizing it completely. That requires us to dismantle and unlearn all of our damaging beliefs about sleep, and *give ourselves permission* to rest, relax, turn in, lie-in, say no to things that will interfere with our sleep, and actually *allow* our minds to switch off.

That's how meditation can help. It teaches us that rest, and by extension sleep, is *just* as important, if not *more* important, than work. They should be scheduled in your calendar just like an important appointment. Because if you don't prioritize rest, your body will do it for you. Maybe a one-off all-nighter might help you finish that project, but if that's your coping strategy forever, it's not going to last too long without serious consequences for your mind and body. (I still associate morning birdsong with university all-nighters and looming essay deadlines, and get a bit of a shudder down my spine despite myself when I hear it now!)

The science shows that getting (on average) at least eight hours' sleep per night will help you:

- Get *more* done, not less, as your brain and bodily functions will operate far more efficiently
- Stop craving crap, and find it easier to fuel your body with healthy nutrition
- Improve your memory

- Feel happier and more clear-headed
- Have more energy
- Improve your immune system, leaving you less vulnerable to ill health, chronic conditions and stress
- Feel better in your own skin
- Improve communication with people around you
- Enhance your relationships
- Increase your feeling of calm, peace and happiness

And yep – you guessed it – mindfulness can also massively help improve your sleep, and helps give you the permission you need to log off, shut down and switch off.

How mindfulness helps sleep

Know thy sleep needs

Because mindfulness helps you to sit with yourself and recognize your patterns, it helps you figure out what works for you, and implement it unapologetically. This is where we can take control of our day, rather than the other way around.

To find out what your sleep pattern is, first, ask yourself these questions:

- When do I feel most awake?
- When does my brain feel most creative and focused?
- If I could sleep without setting an alarm, when would I wake up?

- If I could work at any time – midday to midnight – when would I prefer?
- What would be my ideal wake-up routine, or night-time routine?
- What habits and patterns do I already have, which I know hinder or help my sleep?
- What realistic, easy things could I do to help myself further, e.g., switching to decaf coffee after 1pm, spraying lavender oil on my pillow, buying a blackout blind, wearing earplugs...?

I'm no sleep scientist, but here are some other steps that I've learned work for me and my clients when we're trying to be more mindful about sleep, and kinder to ourselves.

They may sound obvious, but often we need a little nudge to do what we already suspect might help.

Hinders sleep	Helps sleep
Watching phone videos until 11pm	Turning your phone on airplane mode at 9pm and putting it out of reach
Drinking caffeinated coffee or tea all day	Switching to decaf or non-caffeine drinks at midday
Not having any night-time routine and falling into bed whenever and however	Setting an alarm on your phone at a good time, having a bath, and reading fiction for five minutes before turning off the light
Using normal bed sheets and standard pillows because you always have	Buying a cosy blanket or extra soft or supportive pillow that feels like a treat

Hinders sleep	Helps sleep
No physical exercise during the day, or exercising too early or too late for your body	Physical exercise when you can, and when feels right for you, even some gentle yoga or a ten-minute walk
Looking at bright screens all day without the night mode on	Turning down the brightness and setting the "night light mode" on your phone and laptop after sunset
Saying "yes" when people suggest 7am deadlines and 9pm meetings	Setting boundaries around when you can work – except in emergencies – and suggesting alternative times when possible
Having bright lights on at home in the evenings until late	Turning down lights or having "the big light off" and using lamps instead when you start to wind down

Ultimately, it's about knowing yourself, being unapologetic about what you need, and building good habits into those five or ten minutes you would otherwise spend scrolling on social media. Set boundaries, and let others know them. Set a reminder on your phone to start winding down at 9:30pm – whatever you have to do. Sleep is a priority, like anything else on your calendar. Treat it that way.

I know from experience that it's not at all easy when you're in a 9-to-5, but even *trying* to align the time that you *do* have to your own internal clock is a good goal. You'll feel so much better for it.

Ditch the guilt

I give you permission to give up the sleep guilt. Despite what our modern "always on" culture says, every single person needs good sleep. It doesn't make you weak, less efficient, lazy, boring, miss out or fall behind. It makes you human. Our brains need it, and our bodies crave it.

One of the more shocking facts related by Walker in his book is that if you drive a car when you have had less than five hours' sleep, you are 4.3 times more likely to be involved in a crash than if you'd slept for longer, and if you drive having had just four hours, that rises to 11.5 times more likely. As he writes: "It is disquieting to learn that vehicular accidents caused by drowsy driving exceed those caused by alcohol and drugs combined."[7]

Learning how to prioritize and get good sleep is actually a *responsible* thing to do, and helps us get ahead (however you define it) in pretty much every single area of our lives. Work, health, fitness, relationships – you name it, pretty much anything will likely be improved by better sleep.

Alexa, switch off my brain

Learning the tools of mindfulness can help us to wind down and switch our racing mind off at night, just as much as they can help us wake up in the mornings... which is great if you're thinking, "OK, I *know* I need to sleep more, but how the *hell* do I do it? My mind spins out of control as soon as my head hits the pillow."

Good news: A slight tweak to the techniques used during our daily meditation sessions can help us to still and calm our minds before and when we hit the hay, too. A regular meditation practice helps us to switch off our mind before we sleep because it trains us to:

• Become aware of our thoughts and feelings, and take a mental step back from them, so we are not consumed by them, and can rest

- Understand which thoughts are helpful, and which amount to unhelpful rumination, so we can stop worrying and sleep
- Learn to put our thoughts aside temporarily and get the rest we need in the meantime
- Know that our minds are always running – it's what they do – and that a busy mind doesn't necessarily mean something is wrong or that we need to "fix" it
- Connect our mind and body so we can focus on relaxing each part of our body in turn, and concentrate on deliberate and calming physical and mental relaxation
- Build compassion for ourselves, and realize that just because there is more on our to-do list or we didn't get it all done today, we still deserve rest, just as a child or any other human would
- Learn that taking time out to recharge will make us more productive and help us feel better in the long run

We can also invoke the tools of mindfulness to ease us into relaxation, and – in contrast to normal meditation, where we're aiming to feel calm but stay alert – allow ourselves to use our breath and body to feel so relaxed and at peace that we fall into a deep, restorative sleep.

If we know that having a busy brain doesn't make us wrong or broken, we are less likely to pile extra shame and worry on top of the stress. Instead, we learn to see our busy mind as a curious, but ultimately normal hazard of having a human brain. We can then treat it with kindness, rather than feeling stressed about feeling stressed, and making ourselves even more tired by worrying about the fact that we can't sleep.

Loving-kindness meditation, where (to summarize) you forgive yourself and everyone else for being human, helps most with this.

You could also try the following exercises:

- Write down tomorrow's priorities the night before, so you know it's all in hand and planned, and there's no need to worry about it right now.
- Keep a notebook by your bed, so that if you do wake up worried or having remembered something, you can make a note.
- Journal a "brain dump" at the end of the day, so you get your worries, and tomorrow's jobs, out on paper, leaving your mind free to sleep.
- Write out a "Handbook of Me". Write a list of things that help when you're burned out or feeling particularly exhausted to remind yourself, even when you're so tired you can't think. Refer to this list and pick something on it when you need a boost.

As usual, I recommend the above with caution, as it's up to you to decide what will work best for you, and what will make you more stressed or less so. But not only is worrying about something incredibly unlikely to help you deal with the situation when it happens, the anxiety of doing so can stop you from getting the mental and physical rest you need to cope and deal with it better. Stopping, resting, getting still and giving yourself permission to stop worrying for a while, will make you *more* productive, effective, energetic and successful – not *less*.

When put like that, it becomes easier to see sleep not as the lazy, time-wasting thing we were taught it was, and more as a healing, restorative and truly responsible thing to do for our minds, bodies and lives. I'll finish this point with one of my favourite quotes from Matthew Walker's book (and let's be honest, there are many): "When sleep is abundant, minds flourish. When it is deficient, they don't."[8]

Now, stop reading this and get some sleep, OK?

MEDITATION TOOL

Body breathing for sleep

Lying down in bed, get into a position that feels comfortable and natural.

Starting with your head and forehead, tense each part of your body in turn. Scrunch it up, tense your muscles, make everything tight. Hold for 2–4 seconds. Then release slowly for 2–4 seconds. Breathe deeply.

Continue down your body: neck muscles, shoulders, back, chest, stomach, arms, hands, hips, legs, feet.

As you relax, allow your muscles to "melt into" the bed or cushion. Breathe, inhaling for three, exhaling for four. Slow down the breaths as you go.

Allow your body to "breathe itself".

Repeat.

10

Mindful Tech

(or, How to Put your Phone Down)

"Instructions for living a life. Pay attention. Be astonished. Tell about it."

Mary Oliver, poet

This chapter starts with me disagreeing with one of the most influential and insightful figures in the meditation community – Andy Puddicombe, the co-founder, face and voice of the major meditation app and company, Headspace.

Let's be clear, when I met him at an event once, I cried with happiness *in front of him* (I can always be relied upon to keep things chill). So I hardly need tell you how much I respect him. But at that same event, he said something that I've now come to completely disagree with (and maybe he has changed his mind too, who knows?). And that's the idea that technology is "neutral", and we *choose* whether or not to engage with it.

I see why he said it. Most of us want to be more mindful around our phones – so why not just, well, do that? Our phone is just a piece of plastic and glass, after all. So if we turn it off or ignore it, it holds no power over us. Simple, right? After all, studies *do* show that putting it in another room helps improve focus and concentration, and every single "detox from your phone" guide recommends stuff such as turning your phone off for periods of time, or keeping it out of your bedroom, in a cupboard or another room.

A study by the University of Texas found that participants who were asked to complete tasks with their phones in another room scored higher when compared to participants who did the same tasks but with their phones placed face-down next to them. Researchers even found that the participants who had their phones face down within reach did worse, because their brains were actively working to *not* pick up the phone. "The mere presence of their smartphone was enough to reduce their cognitive capacity."[1] So when it comes to our devices, the idea that "out of sight is out of mind" isn't entirely false.

Newsflash: you are a "user" of tech

For years I believed that our phones are neutral, and it's up to us to control how we use them. But then, I spoke to Liza Kindred, a trained meditation teacher, mindful tech expert, and founder of the excellently named Eff This!

meditation community. Speaking on my podcast, she flat-out told me:

> *"Technology is not neutral. It may have been at one point, but that's not true anymore. We have companies making decisions that are really harming us. This is not about [your phone use being] a personal character flaw... or exerting more willpower.*
>
> *"Your phone may be a piece of glass and plastic if it's turned off. But when your phone is turned on, you have a lot of algorithms that are being specifically designed to be addictive. There are literal scientists in labs trying to figure out how to make technology more addictive."[2]*

In the past few years, this idea that our technology is not neutral, but is in fact designed to be utterly distracting and addictive, has become more compelling. The 2020 Netflix documentary *The Social Dilemma*, which explores "the dangerous human impact of social networking", reminds us of a chilling quote from statistician Edward Tufte: "There are only two industries that call their customers 'users': illegal drugs and software."[3] And, as with illegal drugs, we have become helplessly and unintentionally addicted.

In 2018, communications regulator Ofcom published a ten-year review of how smartphones have changed people's lives in the UK, since they first "took off" in 2008. It found that 95% of 16–24-year-olds now have a smartphone, and that "People in the UK now check their smartphones, on average, every 12 minutes of the waking day." It found that 65% of adults under the age of 35 look at their phone within five minutes of waking up, and 60% do so in the five minutes before lights out.[4] And in the US, a separate study found that 47% of smartphone users say they "couldn't live without their devices".[5]

The damaging effects of addictive tech

Now, I don't know about you, but checking your smartphone every 12 minutes – which seems like quite a long gap to me, actually! – and feeling as though I "can't live" without my phone, doesn't exactly chime with my desire to be a mindful, productive, calm and happy person. To me, it sounds a lot like *mindlessness,* or reaching for something out of habit or comfort, rather than due to necessity or genuine interest.

And a 2016 review of available research on the topic, published in the journal *Front Psychiatry*, revealed that several personality traits and conditions were associated with problematic phone use, including low self-esteem, anxiety and depression.[6] While it's not clear whether smartphone use was causing the problem, or that people who suffer from these issues are more likely to reach for their phone, either way, it's evident that the issues are linked.

The NHS defines addiction as "not having control over doing, taking or using something to the point where it could be harmful to you",[7] which anyone who has ever struggled to stop scrolling through Instagram long after they've stopped feeling inspired and started feeling like crap, will recognize. And social media is just the start. With email, work, communication, entertainment, reading, shopping, and even friendships and social events increasingly taking place through screens, it's no surprise that so many of us feel addicted to our phones, craving digital detox, and feeling anxious AF. In the UK, there's even a "Digital Detox Cabin" by a company called Unplugged, where you're invited to stay in an off-grid hut in rural Essex, during which they literally *lock up* your smartphone so you can't use it.

Another testimony from *The Social Dilemma*:

> "Our attention is the product being sold to advertisers... Social media isn't just a tool that's waiting to be used. It has its own goals, and it has its own means of pursuing them... Social media starts to dig deeper and deeper down into the brain stem and take over [our] sense of self-worth and identity."[8]

It's clear: Technology's major goal is to steal our attention, distract us to despair, force us to participate publicly in order to feel that we exist, sell us something to scratch that existential itch, and start the cycle all over again, so we feel worse and worse and worse.

In her book *How To Do Nothing*, Jenny Odell explains why it's so important to "resist the attention economy".[9] She tells the history of "getting away from it all", from giving up mainstream society altogether to her highly relatable fantasy of wanting to throw her phone into the sea.

And she's not alone. Since 2004, the number of people Googling "digital detox" has skyrocketed, peaking in September 2020, just over half a year after the COVID-19 crisis forced millions to stay at home and rely on screens more than ever.[10] That's not necessarily a bad thing in itself, but it does make the issue of digital addiction, and the downsides of tech overuse, even more apparent.

Our *attention* is now big business – a valuable commodity – and if we want to maintain control of our mental health, it makes sense to be wise about where and how we pay that attention.

Reclaiming your mind

Some respond to this intense digital pressure by going the other way, and declining to use social media at all. My partner doesn't, and it took one of my best friends almost a decade to get an iPhone after I first bought mine.

But for many of us, digital balance is a tightrope-walk. It almost goes without saying that the internet, social media and smartphones can be wonderful. I barely know how to do life without it – from booking a flight, to chatting to friends, to listening to music – nor would I make any money if I switched it all off tomorrow, as my career is almost entirely online.

And before we swear off phones completely, we would do well to remember that the internet played a central role in movements such as the Arab Spring in 2010–2012; and in 2021, the UN began gathering smartphone footage to investigate possible crimes against humanity by police and soldiers after the coup in Myanmar – something that would never have been possible before the advent and widespread accessibility of digital devices.[11] Beyond that, remarkable technological innovations using smartphones and mobile apps are providing lifesaving, life-changing improvements to people all over the world in almost every sector you can think of. It would be a mistake – and a marker of enormous privilege – to suggest we should give up our devices forever.

In fact, *not* being on social media is already a luxury reserved for the very few. Only people who don't need the extra attention, exposure, insight, money or connection – such as already-famous actors or already-successful entrepreneurs – have the freedom to never post a single photo or hashtag, or only check their email once a week. Most of us mere mortals cannot and aren't going to give up technology altogether. So, what to do?

I believe the solution is – in the words of my Buddhist teacher Lodro Rinzler in his 2021 book of the same name – to learn to "take back your mind".[12] Our goal here is not to ignore or deny the technology that has become so central to our lives and our world. It's not to turn back the clock and pretend that email, smartphones, social media, newsfeeds and the internet don't exist. Instead, it's to wrest our attention *back* from all of that, so we can live alongside it, without completely losing ourselves.

When I spoke to Lodro on my podcast, he explained the link between constant distraction, news consumption, social media and technology use, and rising and persistent levels of anxiety and stress – and how meditation helps. He said:

"Anxiety is the other epidemic [as opposed to COVID-19] that we don't talk about. Now is the time to ask: How can we take back our mind?... Social media boosts our comparing mind and makes us feel less than whoever we're looking at. Even though of course, they're doing the same thing.

"The idea for [my] book was hatched before [the] pandemic began. But now, we are living through what may be the most universally anxious time of our life. But there are always going to be stressors. Do we want to lock ourselves in a state of anxiety around that stressor? Or do we want to say 'No, I can acknowledge that I can come back to the present moment?'"

Crucially, this doesn't mean ignoring the reality of the situation. As Lodro says,

"People say, 'No, Lodro, you don't understand; rent is due. I don't have the money in the bank. I need to deal with that.' Of course, there are real world problems. But we can address it. We can say, 'OK, here's the time I'm going to do it,' as opposed to, 'I'm going be anxious every moment between now and when I pay the rent'. I could choose to address the situation, or I can choose to freak myself out about it."[13]

Training in meditation and mindfulness is a major way we can do this. It helps us to train our attention, choose where we want to put it and don't, and treat whatever we find there with compassion. And that's exactly the tonic we need after a long day of "doomscrolling" – the word, incidentally, that the New Zealand Public Address chose as its "Word of the Year 2020", to describe "the act of consuming a large quantity of negative online news at once".[14]

Practical steps

I've found the following practices useful in my own life for more mindful tech use:

- Turning off notifications and sounds.
- Deleting news apps and notifications.
- Switching on airplane mode after 9pm.
- Turning on "Do Not Disturb" mode between 9pm and 8am.
- Moving apps to different screens to make them harder to open.
- Moving apps around so I don't know where they are; that extra split second of searching allows me to think: "Do I really want to look at this, or am I just distracted/doing it out or habit?"
- Deleting apps I haven't used for a while.
- Deleting apps when they get too distracting and negative (Twitter and Instagram, I'm looking at you).
- Not using social media at the weekends or in the evenings, and sometimes for longer.
- Putting my phone out of easy reach when I'm in bed.
- Turning my phone face-down when I'm eating/working.
- Leaving my phone in another room whenever possible.
- Filling my phone with apps that support my goals, such as guided meditations.
- Asking myself what I'm really looking for when I pick up my phone. Am I bored? Distracted? Hungry? Avoiding work? Do I need a hug? A stretch? Sleep? – and doing that instead.

And establishing a meditation practice is a great way to help break our addiction to technology. By training our brain to be more mindful, we become more focused, less distracted and look externally to fill a void less often. As a result, we can use our devices as they were originally intended: as tools that make our life better and easier, rather than a digital treadmill on which we must endlessly run, like a sad, selfie-taking lab rat with an Instagram account.

MEDITATION TOOL

Interrupting automatic habits

Sit in meditation, with your phone within reach. If you like, close your eyes.

Notice your breath. Relax your shoulders.

Imagine your phone, sitting there. Notice any urges to reach for it, but don't do it. Why do you want to? What are you searching for? Notice the physical sensations and thoughts that come up. Is it just habit? Are you bored? Worried? Anxious?

How do the feelings change as you continue to breathe? Imagine your phone is now off, or in another room. Does that change anything? Be curious.

Breathe. Repeat.

11

Meditation for
Body Confidence

(or, How to Feel Better about the Skin You're In)

*"Imagine if we all stopped expending so much energy
on trying to change our bodies. We could do anything
we dreamed of. We could get shit done."*

Megan Jayne Crabbe, writer and influencer @bodyposipanda

Body image is the final frontier for many women, myself
included. I'm a victim of what I know now to be largely
bullshit diet culture, and internalized fat phobia toward
myself. And it sucks. For years, I've hated my short, "cute",
"chubby" body for not looking the way I think it should –
and have been on some kind of diet (or felt guilty about
food) all my adult life.

It's been a lifelong and still-ongoing journey to unlearn all
the bullshit beliefs I've grown up with as a "not skinny" woman

in a culture that worships thinness... and even though I adore body positive Instagrammers for their glorious colourful outfits and unapologetic curves, when it comes to myself, I have always struggled to accept my body as it is.

Despite working on my self-worth for years, I still have a long list of items of clothing I would never wear in public. Taking my cardigan off on a hot day sometimes feels like a revolutionary act, and there are many photos of me out there that still bring hot shame when I see them. If you're a woman whose body does not conform 100% to society's ideals, you might relate to this.

The way I look physically has had a definite negative impact on my confidence: my self-belief, what I wear, how I show up, how I compare myself to other people, and how much I believe I deserve to exist. I've often wondered whether I'm pretty, sexy, thin, attractive or beautiful enough to speak up, be loud, show up and have confidence in myself.

Of course, as the "good student" I am, I've long tried to "take control", and have tried pretty much every diet and exercise fad going: Keto, Atkins™, the Whole30® Program, intermittent fasting, 1,200 calories a day, HIIT, weight-lifting, macros, juicing, green smoothies, intuitive eating, cutting carbs, Low GI, eating carbs only once a day, eating only when I'm hungry, eating plant-based, eating whatever I want, etc, etc. But none of it "worked" or made me happy – even if I *did* lose weight for a while, before it all piled back on – because until recently, I never realized that what I *actually* needed to lose was the negative voice inside my head.

We are what we think

Body confidence is not 100% about how we look. It's also about how we talk to ourselves about our body, on the inside. It's about whether we think our body deserves to be loved and respected exactly how it (she?) is. Not when she loses 20lbs, but right now. We need to work on our internal voices first.

That's where meditation shines. It helps us to examine those beliefs about ourselves, to remember that *we cannot hate ourselves into sustainable change*. Remember that awful running coach I spoke about in an earlier chapter? His shouting may have got you moving... but it was the kind, encouraging, compassionate coach who got results. Personally, the only time I have *ever* had any success with long-term healthy changes in my body – such as regular yoga, running and walking, eating in a balanced, relaxed way without guilt, deprivation or shame – is if I am motivated by:

- Love for myself as I am now
- Self-respect for my body
- Wanting to feel healthier and happier

Notice that list does not include self-hatred, self-loathing or a desire to be smaller. If I want to eat something that is perhaps less nutritious (notice I do not say "good" or "bad" – there's no judgement here), if I want to skip a workout, or can feel myself listing everything I think is wrong with my body as I stand in front of the mirror after a shower, I try to think:

- Is this helpful?
- Is this true?
- Is this a good use of my mental energy and time?
- Is this loving and respecting my body, or damaging it and bringing me down?
- Are these my usual self-hatred patterns showing up?
- Did I feel OK yesterday and feel crap today, therefore proving it's all in my head?
- Will this make me feel better or worse?
- Is there another kinder, happier way I could think about this?
- Will this train of thought take me closer to – or further away from – the person I want to be?
- Could I be grateful for my body instead?
- Could I just not hate it? How about that?

It's so much easier to do the right thing for yourself when you're aligning your inner voice with that kind, balanced, nourishing state, rather than deferring to denial and self-hatred. Love wins, always – and never more so than when it's love for yourself.

Inner critic versus utterly systemic

But this isn't where I tell you to just "love yourself", and send you off on your way. The issue is much deeper than that. Body self-hatred – like so many other forms of lack of self-worth – is an issue with our internal narrative, *and* it's systemic. Our internal narratives about the way we look, the way others look and the way we think we "should" look do not exist in a vacuum. They are interconnected, and wrapped up in issues of gender, race and capitalism. It's not our fault we absorb these messages about how we think we should look – it's the culture we live in.

As much as I – a short, rounded white woman – feel ill-at-ease in society, I imagine that state has the potential to be harder still for so many others. We all carry our own difference heavily in a world that sees only thin, white, tall, able-bodied beauty as the perfect ideal.

And just as meditation is a technique to help us deal with the voices inside our own heads, it is also a tool to help us address what's going on *outside* our heads too, to examine where those voices come from in the first place, and then try to change them (see Chapter 15 for more). To paraphrase the story by David Foster Wallace: "A goldfish doesn't know it's in water."[1] As women, we're swimming in the toxic, patriarchal, capitalist water of our society, with messages saying that women must look good and be attractive to men and/or according to some imagined standard.

We don't even realize that this is obscuring our view of who we really are. Which is exactly why this book needs a chapter on body image, despite my feeling unqualified to write it. Because I, as much as anyone, still need to practise applying the lessons of self-compassion, perspective, compassion for others, and activism that meditation and mindfulness can teach us. "Radical self-compassion" is not just a nice concept. It's utterly necessary in a culture that seeks to erase women who do not fit into its narrow mould. And I'm here to help us – you AND me – do it together, the best way I know how.

As Megan Jayne Crabbe, the body positivity campaigner and writer known on Instagram as @bodyposipanda, writes in her book *Body Positive Power: How Learning to Love Yourself Will Save Your Life:*

> *"Hating our bodies is something that we learn, and it sure as hell is something that we can unlearn... We can't see the beauty in everything that we are, because we've been taught to first see everything that we're not."[2]*

Playing small

And body image is not just about having the "perfect" hair, skin, nails or dress size. It's also about how we show up in the world, how we see ourselves in public. Whether we – in the words of the author Tara Mohr – "play big"[3] or play small.

At my lowest moments, the desire to make myself smaller, literally, is never more apparent. One day, years ago, during a particularly difficult time, I went into my then-office and had to fight a strong urge to crawl under the desk, curl into a small ball and weep. I wanted to make myself as tiny as possible, as though the smaller I was, the less it would hurt. I wanted to make my body look the way I felt inside.

Even now, when my depression is bad, I want to lie on the floor. I want to "play small" so I don't have to show up in the world, take risks or open myself up to being even more vulnerable. On a wider scale, the same thing happens in society at large. Women are expected to stay small – to be quiet, neat, nice, polite, slender and cute.

The science bears this out. A University of Pennsylvania study found that obese people are routinely seen as being "lazy, incompetent, unattractive, lacking willpower and to blame for their excess weight";[4] while in 2016, researchers at the University of Exeter concluded that a woman who was a stone heavier than a slimmer woman of her same height would earn on average up to £1,500 less per year.[5] And in 2014, a study by Vanderbilt University in Nashville found that overweight women earn less money than slimmer women, but there was little difference in pay between obese men and slim men.[6] In 2017, Tam Fry, from the National Obesity Forum, told the *Guardian* newspaper:

"Overweight women suffer far more than overweight men because people think women should be slim and attractive."[7]

In the same piece, psychotherapist Susie Orbach, author of *Bodies and Fat is a Feminist Issue*, said,

"Men are meant to be big and strong, and women are meant to be tiny and not take up too much space... They can have everything in the world now, but they [still] have to be slim."[8]

It gets worse. Advertising traditionally seeks to erase women, not just to the point where we're all thin and beautiful, but so much so that we barely even exist. We can now whiten, pluck, slim, cover, tone, stretch, blur, hide, cover, contour, shape, mask, "flatter" – you name it – ourselves into submission in the name of beauty. The overall impression is that we are too much as we are, and need to transform our natural state into something refined and acceptable. "Women! Be bold and brave! But not big! And not too loud! Definitely not like that!"

Know your worth

Body image isn't just about the dress size you wear, or me feeling a bit crap about having chubby arms. It's also about knowing our worth in the world. It's about having *the right to show up exactly as we are.* That's one of the reasons why power poses are so damn powerful! As the social psychologist Amy Cuddy says in her famous TED Talk based on her long-term research on body position and posture, "Our bodies change our minds, our minds can change our behaviour, and our behaviour can change our outcomes."[9]

This rings true in my mindfulness work, too. In workshops, on client calls, in my podcast interviews, when I ask women what "being a badass" means to them, it's usually some variation of: "Take up space. Be yourself. Be unapologetic. Walk into a room and be bold. Say what you want. Show up and be yourself. Be big. Be you."

Figuring out and confronting our own body image demons – whether we're talking about dress size or our ability to move in the world how we want – is important. Because, even if – thanks to writer Susan Cain's amazing work on the power of introverts[10] – we may not all need to shout the loudest to be heard anymore, we do still need to *show up* to be counted. And we can't show up – give that presentation, have that tough conversation, stand on that TEDx stage, command authority in our business, do that Instagram Live or record that advertising video for our new product or service – if we're paralyzed by fear about how we look and feel.

That doesn't mean we have to totally love ourselves before we get started. And I'm not dismissing anyone's insecurities as insignificant or easy to change. I mean, fuck, if I had to wait until I *loved* my appearance before I showed up in my business and life, I'd never do anything except sit on the sofa, saying nothing. But life is short, and our goal is to show up in the world and do good shit, yes?

So rather than working toward an endlessly joyful opinion on the state of our body, I prefer to use the tools of meditation and mindfulness to gain a good dose of realistic, helpful, practical wisdom – to help us put two fingers up to the patriarchal norms that would keep us in boxes and high-control underwear – and *show up as we are*, even if we don't love what we see. I mean, I don't *think* the Buddha was talking to women with Instagram accounts when he laid down the sutras (Buddhist scriptures), but heck if meditation doesn't have something to teach us about it all.

Acceptance and body neutrality

I've said it before and I'll say it again: meditation is, above all, a journey of learning to accept yourself, as you are, beneath all the noise and distractions of the outside world. Even if it feels next to impossible. That's the practice.

What we need is self-compassion (see Chapter 4). Remember, the definition of mindfulness is "paying attention, in the present moment, on purpose, without judgement". That means being completely aware of all the negative stories you tell yourself about everything you hate about yourself, and seeing them for what they are: toxic, bitchy, unhelpful bullshit.

But it's also about seeing those stories and not chastising yourself for telling them. It's about recognizing that we are but goldfish in that crappy water. Once you realize you're in that water, you can't unsee it. It's not easy to escape, though. After decades of self-hatred and internalized toxic messages compounded by advertising and social media, it's OK if it takes you a few years to unlearn it all.

That's why I would always advise aiming for "body neutrality" first, rather than instant "self-love". I don't pretend to stand among the body-positive bloggers and influencers online, but I do know that the day I discovered the idea of #bodyneutrality and #bodypositivity, the way I looked at my body and my life improved tenfold. It felt almost exactly like the day I discovered meditation and mindfulness. Finally, here was a message that made sense. Suddenly, I didn't have to *love my body* overnight, and I didn't have to want to dance around in my pants in public.

I could just be who I was, in my own body, and be OK with it. Body neutrality means you don't have to be super positive, or pretend to know all the answers. As with meditation, you can learn to replace all that inner noise and self-hatred with a sort of peaceful, quiet disinterest. What a relief!

You might actually use that mental energy to do something enjoyable, fun, productive – *anything* else – without being constantly held back by that inner voice that tells you that you're too fat, short, tall, awkward, ugly… whatever. Neutrality means that you can get curious about how mean you are being to yourself, and investigate all the reasons why and how you started talking to yourself like that in the first place, without adding any more shame or judgement.

This is *exactly* what we are trying to do with meditation, and why it's such a powerful tool. It trains our brain to get curious, be interested, question old patterns, and see them for the stories and lies they are. That's why it works in perfect parallel to any quest toward body love and appearance acceptance. Once we don't hate our body, and when we've learned how to mindfully get the perspective and self-acceptance that we need, maybe we might now have the mental and physical space and energy to finally begin to like (or even *love!*) our own beautiful, precious, body.

We are not alone

As loving-kindness mediation teaches us, we're all human, and we all struggle. When we learn to see our body hatred for the toxic BS it is, we can understand the pain that others may be going through about *their* hang-ups, too. It gives us perspective, and when you're drowning in self-hatred, that's a bloody good thing.

I have a memory of being on a beach in Thailand with a friend a few years ago. We'd dressed up a bit after days of zero make-up, and wanted to capture the moment with a photo. I snapped a few, thought we looked fine, and expected to enjoy our dinner out. But what followed was a tedious 20 minutes of my friend directing me in an attempt to capture her "best side" so she'd be able to show everyone back home what a great time she was having. By which time, we'd missed the sunset and I was hungry, bored and annoyed. I just wanted to eat my Thai green prawns and listen to the waves. I could pretend I was above such posing. But no. What *really* bothered me was that I thought my friend looked perfect. I wanted to have her long legs and thin chin, and look like her in photos; and I was miffed she didn't appreciate what she had. It was a reminder, if ever I needed one, that literally everyone has hang-ups we have no idea about. It's really, *really*, not just us.

Another time, I was at a networking event when one totally gorgeous *glamazon* – all bronzed skin, long legs and cheekbones – confessed that she'd stopped posting to her half a million Instagram followers (casual), because she had started hating her face, and was wondering if she needed lip fillers. I almost spat out my Champagne. Here I was, feeling like a troll next to her, and she was fretting about her face.

This constant judging of looks and surprise at others' insecurities also reminds us of how internal and subjective *our* insecurities about our appearance are – and how much others struggle, too. Maybe – maybe! – it's not about the so-called "flaws" of our outside appearance at all?

The more we practise compassion for ourselves, and the more accepting, loving and forgiving we can be toward our own hang-ups, the more we can see that others are suffering from body image issues too. We can recognize that no-one – no matter how perfect or incredible they look – has it all together.

As women, it's ridiculously easy to fall back on the story that the smaller we are, the more we deprive ourselves, the better and more disciplined and more worthy of being loved we are. But when it comes to actual appearance and dress size, I've very quickly found something else to be unhappy about. Yes, I've felt strong, athletic and powerful when I've been eating healthily with good nutrition, or I've run a certain distance, or lifted a certain weight. But, as much as I hate to admit it, my life would not suddenly be perfect if I was a size 4. I know this, because when I *have* managed to lose a few dress sizes off the back of some random diet, it has changed almost *nothing* about my inner chatter. Yes, I've felt good about myself, and sexy, and accomplished, and disciplined, and healthy. But those things are not a size – they're a mindset. And let's not forget the millions of people without the body privilege that I have, who can't just change their body shape or outward appearance with the latest fitness plan.

I can't pretend to talk for anyone else, but I can say, "Hey, *you!* You exist, and you're worthy of taking up space, no matter how you think you look." If Buddhism and mindfulness has taught me one thing, it's that we all have inherent, basic goodness. We are all worthy, and we all deserve to exist, just because we're human. As the Buddhist nun Pema Chödrön rather poetically writes, "You are the sky. Everything else – it's just the weather."[11]

So the key is not to focus too much on changing our external appearance. We all have things we don't like about ourselves, things that don't "fit in" or aren't "right" – some more visible than others, some more damaging and risky than others – and we always will. And for some it can be downright dangerous to exist in the world as they appear. Data from the UK Office for National Statistics found that trans people, for example, are twice as likely to be victims of crime than cisgender people.[12] Talk about being afraid to show up as your real self.

To me, finding body confidence as we are is about changing the inner conversation we have with ourselves about our bodies and our insecurities, *and also* trying to change perceptions in the world around us so that we can all feel comfortable to show up in the world, however we look. Because feeling confident isn't only about changing our inner voice – it's about changing the culture we're swimming in, too. We're all goldfish in a toxic bowl, but we don't need to accept the water – we need to change the entire damn bowl. And meditation is central to that process, helping us move from hatred to acceptance, to love, to compassion, to activism, to real change.

MEDITATION TOOL

Visualization for self-worth

Seated comfortably, imagine that a really good friend or loved one – someone who makes you smile when you think of them – is sitting in front of you.

Visualize them, imagine all the good things about them, the good times you've shared, the ways they're really trying their best, the things they've struggled with but overcome, and all the times they've been a friend to you in the past.

Now imagine telling them that, despite all of that, they're not good enough. They're useless. They don't look right, they're too stupid or too much or just not right, and they're a disappointment to everyone. Imagine telling them that they will never achieve what they want, and that, secretly, everyone judges them, hates them and thinks they're a waste of space.

How does saying all of that to them make you feel? Notice any physical sensations or thoughts.

It's probably not great, right? Downright hurtful and rude and unhelpful, in fact. Maybe you feel as though you want to come to their defence, or you feel terrible for even thinking it.

But each time we talk to ourselves in this way, we're saying those kinds of words to ourselves. And much worse.

Now imagine that you've switched places with your friend, feeling what they feel, after having those things said to them by a friend.

What do you notice? What thoughts and feelings emerge? Does anything surprise you? Do you find yourself making excuses, or thinking it's OK for you to feel that, but not them? Why or why not?

The goal here is to notice what emotions and feelings come up, and ultimately recognise that we can replace them with a kinder, more helpful way of speaking to ourselves.

12

Mindful Self-care

(or, Eating, Drinking and Moving Your Body a Bit)

"We don't meditate to get better at meditating; we meditate to get better at life."

Sharon Salzberg, author and world-renowned meditation teacher

You might wonder why I'm so adamant that being "bad at" meditation means you're doing it right. It's precisely because meditation itself isn't the wider goal. The goal is to take what we learn "on the cushion", as the saying goes, and bring it "off the cushion", into our real life – to practise that focus, and become more mindful generally.

This can feel impossible at first. People struggle to meditate even when they're sitting still – so how the heck are they supposed to bring it into the rest of their life, too? The key is practice. The more we meditate, the less likely we are to totally forget everything as soon as the session ends, and we will become more mindful in our everyday life. In fact, many people find this an easier "way in" to meditation than the pure, sitting-on-the-cushion approach. If you've ever thought: "I don't meditate, but I do paint/run/tidy mindfully", then you'll know what I mean.

And while I don't 100% agree that doing something mindfully and *formally* meditating are the same (studies show that it's the formal sitting-on-the-cushion meditation that makes the biggest brain changes), if you're being more mindful in your everyday life, then that's still a win, I reckon. And it's even more powerful if you're managing to squeeze in a daily meditation session too. A combination of both is best.

Luckily, there are a few ways that we can practise mindfulness in our everyday lives to help us apply the principles we aim for *on* the cushion, *off* it, too. The easiest of these are mindful eating and drinking and mindful movement.

Mindful eating and drinking

If you've ever taken a beginner's meditation course, it's likely you'll have been introduced to the ins and outs of a raisin. It's a classic mindfulness exercise to give someone a raisin, and ask them to notice the texture, smell, colour, taste. Any associations and memories? How it feels to chew, to eat. Temperature, feel, aftertaste. Longing for more?

Through this, we're invited to notice sensations we'd usually miss (by popping the raisin into our mouth without thinking), and therefore see – in theory, anyway – how much richer every single moment of our lives could be, if we only paid attention.

Naturally, in my classes, I use chocolate instead of raisins (tastes better and melts more quickly), but the point is that food can be a great way to practise mindfulness, because of its potential to engage our senses, and the fact that it's remarkably easy to eat food mindlessly.

Taking time to notice each bite of our lunch, rather than scoffing it while we reply to emails; savouring each sip of wine, rather than inhaling a glass over Netflix – can help us tune in to our body and mind and also help us enjoy the food and drink more, too.

Healing our relationship with food and drink

But "mindful eating or drinking" is not just about the physical act. Paying attention to how, when and why we eat or drink can also be an act of self-respect – and a powerful tool in figuring out complex emotions. For many of us, food and drink are tied to our emotions – positive and negative.

Depending on our society and background, food and drink can be a major source of comfort, ritual, love, family, sharing, support, friendship, socializing and more. We eat cake to celebrate. We drink wine to relax. We bake cookies to cheer ourselves up. We drink cocktails to socialize. We attach meaning to food, and we weave stories about when, how, why and *if* we should have it.

But for many of us, these beliefs and cultural expectations around food and drink can tip over into dependency, lack of control and addiction. Many of us wish we could eat less, or eat more healthily, give up sugar, eat less chocolate, drink less wine, or give them up completely. Many of us stop eating well in times of stress, or feel out of control when it comes to food and drink.

Here, too, mindfulness helps. In fact, a 2019 study in the *British Medical Journal* found that mindfulness practices "produce improvements in depressive symptoms... [and] control with respect to eating behaviours in patients", and that "Mental awareness plays an important role in eating behaviour."[1]

And a 2012 study in *the Journal of American College Health* found that "mindfulness was related to healthier eating practices, better quality of sleep, and better physical health".[2] Similarly, psychologist Jean Kristeller found that mindful eating techniques helped reduce participants' "bingeing and depression", and that "mindfulness-based therapy [also] seemed to help people enjoy their food more and have less sense of struggle about controlling their eating."[3]

Of course, mindfulness is not a replacement for therapy or for getting specialist help for addiction, but I'm living proof that being more mindful can help to unravel a lot of the issues so many of us have around food and drink, and help us to take a more measured and sensitive approach to why we eat and drink as we do.

A caveat: "Mindful eating" is sometimes seen as a synonym for "dieting", as in, "eating mindfully" means eating less, and becoming a "perfect person" who always chooses the saintly green salad instead of the "bad", creamy pasta. I'm not about that. As psychologist Joseph B. Nelson wrote: "The purpose of mindful eating is not to lose weight...The intention is to help individuals savour the moment and the food, and encourage their full presence for the eating experience."[4]

While mindful eating helps you change your habits, it's much less about dieting as it is about being respectful of your body, tuning in to what it needs, and what feels good – in the short-term and the long-term – and choosing the best thing for you in that moment. For some, that might be to have a Virgin Mojito instead of a normal one. For others, it might mean eating the chocolate cake. It often makes *perfect sense* to comfort eat when you're seeking comfort.

But, as ever, practising meditation helps you get in touch with your body, and how your emotions and thoughts affect your physical cravings and needs. If we're learning to treat our bodies from a place of respect, and know that we're good enough as we are – no shame needed – then we can get perspective on why, how or when we eat or drink as we do. While this might not fix our addiction to Jaffa Cakes (just me?), it might rein it in a bit, and help us practise more moderation, if we want to. It can stop us from using food or drink as an emotional crutch, whether that means eating *more* food to nourish our body in difficult times, or holding back on using the chocolate eclairs as a coping mechanism.

This doesn't mean that you'll never want to inhale a packet of chocolate chip cookies or an entire bottle of wine in one sitting again (or, conversely, forget to eat when life gets stressful). It just means that if or when you do, you might be more aware why you're doing it. You might feel more in control, and stop at half a pack or a couple of glasses, or replace the behaviour with something healthier, if you want to, without hating yourself.

And, if you're anything like me, you might be able to see that, in those times, your food habits are signalling something deeper. Maybe what you actually need is a nap, a hug, a chat, a therapist, a glass of water or a walk instead. In this way, we can heal our relationship with our body through respect, not self-hatred.

Talking of walks…

Mindful movement

The term "mindfulness" suggests it's solely about the mind. But mindfulness is *also* about the body.

It's also about the benefits of moving more, preferably outside. In fact, I reckon mindfulness could be called "mind-and-bodyfulness" (catchy, eh?), because one of the most important aspects of mindfulness is developing our ability to "drop" into our bodies, and our physical sensations.

As I explained earlier, the connection between mental and physical health, and how we store trauma in our body, is now widely recognized. This "mind-body connection" idea might sound a little "woo" to some, but it's actually not that weird. We're used to the idea that feeling embarrassed means we blush, or we get "butterflies in our stomach" when we're nervous. This is the same thing. Mindfulness teaches us that we can use our mind to become more aware of our body, and vice versa.

In fact, there's no real need for me to make up such a terrible word as "mind-and-bodyfulness", because a word already exists: "embodiment". Loosely speaking, in this context, embodiment means being aware of your body, and understanding how its physical sensations, position and movement are connected to your mind and thoughts.

The meditation teacher Joseph Goldstein has a brilliant phrase he uses to help us "zone in" to our bodies in this way: "Sit, and know you're sitting." How do you know you're sitting? And what can you *feel*? Not the thoughts that come to mind – but what, *physically*, can you feel? How do certain thoughts make certain areas of your body feel? Consider the temperature, texture, tension, aches, looseness, tingling, how it feels from the *inside*. *This* is mindfulness of the body.

Sometimes you don't even need to define these feelings with words. Our brains can, with practice, *feel* something without language. For those of us who feel like we always have to know the answer, this can be a relief. In a world filled with loud opinions and hot takes, knowing that you can process something purely through feeling, without words, can be a relief indeed. Long story short, mindfulness helps us use the body as a powerful tool to ease our frazzled minds.

Get outside

Often, mindfulness also connects awareness of our body with awareness of nature, and the benefits of being outside. There's a reason why the guided meditations I make for my clients often include images such as hiking in nature, trees, waterfalls and streams. In Japan, the mental health benefits of being outside are widely respected. The practice of *shinrin-yoku* (森林浴) – or "forest bathing" – literally means getting outside to connect to nature with all our senses. Studies have shown that it can be considered as a form of nature therapy, and can reduce blood pressure, depression, fatigue and anxiety.[5]

This is, I reckon, one of the reasons why activities such as mindful walking and gardening – activities that combine our need for movement with the peace of being outside – have become so popular in recent years. As Kendall Platt, a mindful gardening coach, who has studied therapeutic horticulture to help people with anxiety and depression, told me:

"Mindful gardening gives you the headspace to be able to grow, and give yourself permission to grow yourself as a person, too.

"There's an element of slowing down, of noticing and engaging all your senses. The feeling of the secateurs in your hand, the sound as you cut through the branch. It's about making the intention to notice what you're doing, and find that calm. Things like mindful seed sowing are great, because it's a very repetitive action.

"Many of the women that come to work with me feel quite disconnected from themselves, and from Mother Nature. They're either working an office job or at home, or [due to COVID] they've been stuck indoors

home-schooling. But actually, it's that connection with Mother Nature and that viewing of the seasons, which are so key. Mindful gardening is a form of rest, which is also outdoors, and active."[6]

Getting outdoors while being active is, basically, the perfect mindful movement equation. As Jonathan Fields writes in his book *Uncertainty*, in celebration of psychiatrist Professor John Ratey's work on exercise and the brain:

"Exercise isn't just about physical health and appearance. It also has a profound effect on your brain chemistry... and neuroplasticity (the ability of the brain to literally rewire itself)... Studies now prove that aerobic exercise both increases the size of the prefrontal cortex and facilitates interaction between it and the amygdala."[7]

And guess what? Those are the *exact* bits of the brain that we're aiming to "improve" when we meditate! Win.

But let me be clear: This isn't me telling you to go for a walk or go outside, and you'll *magically* feel better. In fact, this oversimplification is so common and can – in many cases – be so unhelpful, that there are thousands of memes mocking it online. A personal dark favourite is a particularly bleak photo of a man lying face down on an old mattress in a garden, with the caption: "When you're depressed, and someone says: 'You should go outside'." A May 2020 article in *Self* magazine even implored: "Please, stop telling me to go for a walk."[8]

It is indeed a trite oversimplification to tell someone who is depressed to "just take a walk" or "go outside", when many depressed people struggle to get out of bed or have a shower. In a similar vein, it's pretty able-ist to suggest that "going for a walk" can cure all ills. Some people can't – what about them? To that, I would say: do what you can, in your own way. I recently worked with a client who was in chronic pain after a serious injury. I never once told her to "Just go for a walk!" It would have been unhelpful and insensitive, and she couldn't have done it anyway. Instead, we worked on physical techniques that didn't rely on specific postures or activity, and used her body as a tool to help with her stress in other ways.

The mental health benefits of Mother Nature

But if you *are* able to, and you're dealing with a low mood or a particularly tough patch of anxiety, there is sometimes nothing better, nothing more head-clearing, than *forcing* yourself – yes, I did say "forcing", but in the most compassionate way possible – to get some air on your face and around your body, even if it's a quick dash to the nearest patch of green.

For many of us chronic overthinkers, who have spent far too many hours in our heads or in front of a computer, getting outside and moving our bodies in a slightly different way can shift our energy in near-miraculous ways. This is annoying as hell, I know. I struggle as much as the next person to get out of the house, especially when work is busy or my anxiety and depression are high. A walk for no reason feels like a waste of time when I've got loads to do, or impossible when I'm feeling so mentally crap that I can barely brush my hair. And there's nothing smugger than someone who goes for a run at 5am, and then proceeds to tell everyone about it for the rest of their life. (I mean, is it even a run if you don't post about it on Instagram? Sigh.)

But, *so many* studies have shown that getting out in nature can be beneficial for our mental health. One 2018 report from the University of East Anglia, which analysed data from 140 studies of 290 million people across the UK, US, Spain, France, Germany, Australia and Japan, found that being close to nature and spending time outside can reduce stress and lower heart rate, among a host of other benefits.[9] Lead author of the study, Caoimhe Twohig-Bennett, told *Science Daily*:

"We found that spending time in, or living close to, natural green spaces is associated with diverse and significant health benefits. In fact, one of the really interesting things we found is that exposure to greenspace significantly reduces people's levels of salivary cortisol – a physiological marker of stress. This is really important because in the UK, 11.7 million working days are lost annually due to stress, depression or anxiety.

"Forest bathing is already popular as a therapy in Japan – with participants spending time in the forest sitting or lying down, or just walking around. Our study shows that perhaps they have the right idea!"[10]

If mindfulness is defined as "paying attention, on purpose, without judgement", then it stands to reason that you can do that outside too, for the dual benefits of nature plus mindfulness (as well as the fitness benefits, if that's your thing). So next time you feel like you need a break, I highly recommend telling yourself to go outside for five minutes.

Maybe try some or all of these techniques as you go:

- Count your steps up to ten, then start again at one.
- Feel the way your feet walk or run, the texture of the ground. Notice how the gravity shifts from one side to the other.
- Notice sounds and smells, such as the birdsong in the trees or smoke in the autumn air.
- Count your breaths as you move.
- Walk to a natural area and allow yourself ten minutes to sit, breathe, meditate and/or notice sounds and scents.
- Zone in on your shoulders and relax them while you jog or walk.
- Count how many different types of leaves or trees you can see.
- Make a note of all the "pinks", "blues", "reds", etc.
- Notice your body. Is your breathing speeding up or slowing down? Any tension or relaxation anywhere? Can you breathe more deeply?

These things may sound ridiculously simple, and frankly boring compared to a good podcast, but even just trying them for five or ten minutes as you step outside for a walk or run, before you put the headphones on, can work wonders for a stressed-out brain. As Bella Mackie writes in her down-to-earth running memoir, *Jog On*:

> *"Running [outside] is not magic beans and I now know that I can't expect it to inure me to the genuine sadness of life. But throughout tough periods in my life, and without realising it, I had finally acquired a coping skill… It's hard to run and feel sorry for yourself at the same time."*[11]

Other excellent writers – from Haruki Murakami to Alexandra Heminsley, to Bryony Gordon – have all written brilliant books about the mental health benefits of running outdoors[12] – whether you fancy marathons or a jog down the street – so I won't repeat their work here. But it's an undeniable fact that getting outside and moving your body in some way is good for you. And being mindful while you're doing it can help you get even more benefits from it.

And even if you can't get outside, studies suggest that we get similar mental health boosts by just *looking at* nature. Happily, a 2015 study in the *Journal of Physiological Anthropology* showed that having a real plant *inside* the house can make you feel more "comfortable, soothed, and natural".[13] A 2007 survey even backed up earlier research that found that having plants in your workspace helps productivity and creativity.[14] All hail the humble house plant!

So if going for a walk or a jog is out of the question or simply feels like too much, maybe a good old kitchen boogie surrounded by your pot plants might help! Turns out that even taking your cup of coffee to a wide-open window might be enough.

EXPLORING EMOTION THROUGH NATURE

Getting closer to nature can also help us to understand and explore our emotions more fully, so we can work through them more effectively. For example, if I ask you how you're feeling, you might not be able to articulate it. But if you tell me that you're feeling your emotions like a waterfall, rushing out of control and smashing onto your head, or that you feel like you're pushing a boulder up a hill, or you feel bleak like it's a rainy day, suddenly I understand what you mean.

Similarly, if you tell me that your mind feels like a clear blue sky or still lake, or your mood is finally improving like the first daffodils waking up after a long winter, that paints a picture better than any over-intellectualized definition of your mental state ever could.

It's why I love using nature metaphors in guided meditations for clients, and why so many respond so strongly to them. I might guide one client through a mountain hiking visualization to help her believe she can reach her goals, or ask another to imagine her thoughts are a waterfall rushing past. The images are obvious to the point of banal, but despite – or because of? – that, they're wildly effective. It's almost enough to make me want to hug a tree.

Tools for embodiment

Learning the tools of "embodiment" can help us show up in the world the way we want to. We can use our newfound physical awareness to not only notice what our brains are doing, but to change our perception of ourselves and of our behaviour through our body. One of my favourite parts of embodiment theory is commonly known as the "four embodiment types". Based on the four elements, they describe how we move in our bodies, and how this connects to personality and behaviour. They are:

Four embodiment types		
Type	**Physical posture**	**Qualities**
Fire	Leaning forward. Ready to go.	Strong. Confident. Powerful. Forceful.
Water	Yielding. Leaning back.	Placid. Thoughtful. Calm.
Air	Hands up. Loose. Flowy.	Spontaneous. Flowing. Casual.
Earth	Straight lines. Rigid. Feet front-facing, shoulders straight.	Steadfast. Reliable. Grounded.

There are tests you can take to see which type fits you best, but you can also feel your way into it by trying each pose in turn, and seeing which feels more natural. (They're not like star signs, so if you're Aquarius, it doesn't mean you'll necessarily be more "Water" here!)

- Which one feels most like you?
- Which one do you think you are in life, usually?

- Imagine yourself in a challenging situation: a job interview, a date, a presentation. How would you want to show up in each?
- Are you usually quite watery and timid, but could do with more of Fire's spark?
- Or are you usually quite earthy and rule-abiding, but would love a bit of Air's spontaneity?

For example, I tend to be quite fiery when I'm working. I'm confident, outspoken and I have no patience for rules or "how things have always been done". That can be great when it comes to speaking up and getting things accomplished, but that same Fire sometimes means I talk more than quieter people, and dismiss proper processes in my bid to blaze ahead.

I've had to work on becoming more Earth to work effectively in a team, and be more Water and yielding, to allow other more timid or quieter colleagues to speak. Similarly, in my relationship, this Fire can be great, making me confident and cheeky. But it can sometimes cause me to be more confrontational or guarded than I want to be. So, with my partner, I might aim to be more watery and airy – open, yielding, softer, spontaneous.

Overall, embodiment is – within this context, anyway – yet another way to get to know ourselves better, and show up more mindfully and intentionally as we are in the world. We need mindfulness to give us the humility and insight to see ourselves for who we are, so we can be aware of our patterns and choose more helpful next steps. We can even channel this through new activities if we really want to make a change.

Activities to challenge embodiment types		
Type	**Wants to be more**	**Try**
Fire	Water	Ballroom dancing where someone else has to lead. Challenge yourself to let others speak first.
Water	Fire	Boxing. Challenge yourself to speak up first, with confidence.
Air	Earth	Power yoga. Figuring out a logic puzzle.
Earth	Air	Going on a journey that someone else has planned and that you don't know any details about.

None of this requires us to be super-fit, or to have the time and energy or ability to go for a long hike, so it's a great way to connect to ourselves physically, as well as mentally – to positive, wide-ranging, long-term and life-changing effect, without needing to have a forest on our doorstep!

MEDITATION TOOL

Feel your feet

When you feel your thoughts spiralling and your anxiety rising, stop. Whether you're standing or sitting, "drop" your attention and focus to your feet, physically.

Tune in your attention to how they feel in your shoes / slippers / socks / bare feet. How is your weight balanced on them? Are they tense? Achy? Warm? Cold? Breathe.

Unlike our mind, which can take us to any number of places in the past or future, our body can only be here, where we are, in this very moment.

Continue to breathe, and imagine that you're breathing into your feet and body, as though it were hollow and expanding, like a balloon.

Drop your shoulders even more. Count your breaths in, then out. Notice how your body responds.

Does anything shift?

13

Meditation for Good Sex and Relationships

(or, Safety, Solitude and Mindful Sex)

"I don't need anyone else to distract me from myself anymore, like I always thought I would."

Charlotte Eriksson, author and songwriter

When it comes to thinking about meditation and sex, your mind might go straight to the Kama Sutra, or you may think that the two must be mutually exclusive, because well, mindfulness equals being Buddhist, wise, and chaste, right? Well, I'm no sexpert, but I know that meditation can absolutely improve your relationships and sex life. How?

Because, as you'll know if you've read this book so far, meditation improves your:

- Self-confidence and the ability to feel safe in your mind
- Body confidence and the ability to feel safe in your body

- Communication, with yourself and others
- Self-belief, and knowing what you want and need (and how to get it)
- Ability to be vulnerable and open
- Ability to be strong and powerful
- Ability to work through trauma and past negative experiences with gentleness
- Ability to be in the present

The more I've learned about mindfulness and meditation, the more I find I am able to put my own needs first, without too much ego or fear, and treat my long-term partner the way I want to be treated, while always having the confidence and self-respect to speak up when I need to. Unsurprisingly, I put much of the success of our relationship down to mindful communication and respect, and a healthy amount of independence – as well as a continued commitment to understanding that there's always more to learn about each other, and always more compassion and respect needed, no matter how long you've been together.

Admittedly, maybe after we've been together for 30 years (only 23 to go!), I'll feel differently. But right now, I am convinced that mindfulness holds a lot of wisdom, not only about knowing ourselves, but also in terms of how we relate to others. This chapter is my take on how it can help us to achieve kinder, deeper, happier, more respectful and more fulfilling relationships.

Before I met my partner, I was going on a different date every week (so many mediocre cocktails). I definitely learned some tips along the way, and realized that my meditation practice was helping me in ways I'd never imagined. Without telling you my entire dating life story, here's what I learned about how meditation helps – whether you're swiping right every day, or simply thinking about dipping your toe back in the pool.

Before we dive in, remember that you bring *so much* to the table just by being you, and you don't need a relationship or a sex life to feel good about yourself – it's just an excellent bonus. With that said, let's do this.

First, a disclaimer

I'm well aware that I've oversimplified a lot of the nuances of dating, relationships and sex in this chapter. Though I hope that this advice can be applicable to everyone, I haven't given any specific advice for people in the LGBTQIA+ communities or people with deeper trauma, discrimination and issues that may affect their confidence and ability in these areas, for example. The main reason for this is that I am very much aware that I'm not the best person to do that, and the other reason is because my editor will kill me if I make this book any longer.

I have tried to give general advice on how to be more mindful in relation to sex and relationships, and I hope you're able to take what makes sense to you from this chapter, and leave the rest, or seek advice from a specialist for more specific help if needs be.

Above all, remember – when it comes to dating, relationships and sex, the most important thing is to keep yourself safe, physically and emotionally. Always tell people where you are, check in with friends, communicate what's happening, and run (physically and digitally) from anyone who makes you feel even a little bit belittled, confused, gaslit, abandoned, mocked, badly treated, shamed, threatened or otherwise unsafe. You're worth so much more.

Dating and relationships: How mindfulness helps

Self-awareness, and unapologetic knowledge of your needs

When I started dating seriously after my last break-up, I was determined and absolutely unashamed in my approach. I went out there with a singular aim: to find someone who wanted a serious relationship. I was looking for someone who was respectful, who I fancied physically, connected with mentally, laughed with, who didn't make dodgy sexist, racist or political jokes, wanted a serious relationship too, and felt the same way about me. I was happy to be super open about this, and no longer felt embarrassed about stating it on my dating profile, and on dates themselves. If anyone showed the slightest sign of playing games, or not meeting even a single one of my criteria, I'd let them know and move on – sharpish.

It worked, and it saved me (and my dates) a lot of time. You won't be surprised to hear that regular meditation helps you to do this – get so acquainted with your own needs, feelings, boundaries and expectations that you no longer accept anything less than you deserve.

Presence, respect and communication

Training your mind to be in the present not only means you enjoy life more, it also makes you a better listener, communicator and partner in general. If you're able to actually *listen* to someone, you can respond better to them.

Listening to someone, remembering what they say, communicating your own interests and needs without second-guessing yourself all the time, are all key parts of great dating. Unsurprisingly, it's much more enjoyable to listen to and respect someone you've just met, than it is to be constantly distracted, worrying about what you're going to say next, doubting yourself, and stressing out about what happens if there's an awkward silence. Be present, breathe and enjoy being yourself.

Good listening also helps the other person feel more appreciated, so you can build a better connection more quickly, and – crucially, on a date – helps you to decide in record time if they're boring you senseless.

Finding safety in solitude

It's a bloody annoying-but-true paradox that the less you need a partner and the better you are at spending time alone, the more likely you are to enjoy being with someone, and to be a better partner yourself.

When you're not totally dependent on someone else to feel entertained or good enough, you can focus on enjoying being with them, and see any time you spend with them as a bonus, rather than something you *need* to feel complete.

There's nothing worse than going on a date thinking that this one has *got* to work or you'll die alone; or going out with someone who you find soul-crushingly dull, just so you're not sitting at home alone of an evening. And we all know how horrendous it is when someone is being really needy toward us. You're not that person. You're great just as you are. And if, through meditation and practising self-compassion, you *know how to remind yourself of that*, then you can show up fully aware of what you bring to the table, advocate for what you want and need, feel comfortable in yourself, and safe in the knowledge that you don't need another person to feel complete.

Meditation is great for that. It's literally a practice of being with and by yourself in near-silence, regularly, being aware of how you're feeling, learning to be OK with it, and being able to soothe yourself without constant distractions or reliance on others. This can save you from a lot of dodgy situations, and means that you'll never accept a mediocre, potentially dangerous hook-up out of a sense of obligation... because you know that going to bed alone is a perfectly acceptable option.

Sex: how mindfulness helps

So, what if dating has gone well and you're getting physical? Meditation's good for that, too.

The ability to be in the present
It's so clichéd as to have become a joke, but these days, we're less likely to say we're lying back "and thinking of England", and

more likely "lying back and thinking of our massive to-do list, how our belly looks in this light, and when we're going to do that giant pile of washing in the corner".

Of course, we're all tired, busy and distracted, but you don't need me to tell you that sex is way less good if you're thinking of a million other things when it's going on. Because mindfulness trains our ability to drag our mind back to the present, it can be a damn good tool for focusing on what's actually happening; you can tune in to the pleasure, the connection and what you like (and don't). For something as sensual as sex, tuning in to the physical sensations – the smell of your partner's neck, the warmth of your body, the temperature of the room – means you're way more likely to enjoy it if you're *present* to it all. (Especially because that pile of washing will still be there when you're done.)

Body-confidence and vulnerability

As someone who has struggled with this my entire adult life, I am acutely aware of how vulnerable it can feel to reveal your body – in all its goose-pimpled, wobbly glory – to your partner. But mindfulness helps us in three major ways here.

The first is that, as I said in the last point, tuning into how things really *feel* means you're way less concerned about how things *look*. Trust me.

Secondly, the kindness and self-compassion that mindfulness teaches means that we are far less likely to be so critical about ourselves, and we will realize that whatever our body looks like, we're still deserving of pleasure, and can learn to enjoy it.

And thirdly, mindfulness helps us to set boundaries on what we do and do not accept – in terms of behaviour from ourselves, and from others. Anyone having sex with you should make you feel sexier and better about yourself and your body, not worse. If they don't, that's on them, not you. Work on loving your body as it is, not changing it for someone else.

Communication, and getting what you want

Good sex with a long-term partner is like one of those chats where you finish each other's sentences, and everything flows. But in order to get to that place, you need to be open and communicative before, during and after sex. This might mean being confident enough to say, "That's not working for me" or "I prefer this!", or to laugh easily when your body makes a funny noise.

To do that, you need to be able to tune in to what you like and need, and be able to ask for it, *and* be attuned to what your partner is thinking, feeling and wanting, too. The more mindful you are, the more likely you are to pick up on those cues, and to communicate openly, without embarrassment or shame, about what's going on and what everyone wants. Happy days (and nights).

Being strong and powerful

Asking for what you want and getting it, especially in a sexual environment, can be empowering AF. Women are so often socialized to be meek or "play hard-to-get" when it comes to sex, that realizing we can lead, know what we want, ask for it and get it – with all the pleasure that implies – can be fantastically freeing.

Because mindfulness helps us work on our own self-worth, inner power and presence, it helps us bring that intentional, deliberate, self-assured version of ourselves to the sheets, and enables us to be the strong, powerful badass we want to be. I've personally never been with a man who doesn't like a confident woman in the bedroom – and beyond that, I can confidently say that if your sexual partner has got issues with your confidence, and is threatened by it (either in the bedroom or out), that's almost certainly a red relationship flag that needs addressing.

MEDITATION TOOL

Scan for sensations

Once seated in meditation, bring your attention to your breath, and notice where in your body you can feel it most. Notice the gravity of your body, keeping you grounded in place, as you sit.

Tune it to physical sensations, scanning gently and bringing your focus down from the top of your head to the tips of your toes. As you go, notice any texture, warmth, tingling, throbbing, discomfort, tension, softness. You don't have to name the sensations as you go – simply practise bringing your attention to your skin and body, and imagine yourself tuning it to every single tiny nerve ending. Sit for a while, noticing.

As you continue to breathe normally, curve your body inwards gently, tucking your head, and bring your hands around you in a protective, bracing posture. How does that feel?

After a few moments, do the opposite. Open your chest, lift your chin, open your arms, turn your hands to the sky, and sink back. How does that feel? What do you notice?

14

Mindfulness and Financial Wellbeing

(or, Money and Mindfucks)

"Money is not the only answer, but it makes a difference."

Barack Obama, 44th president of the United States

I am far from an expert on money, but I do know that it can be a total mindfuck, *especially* if you're ambitious, with a "side hustle" or your own business. That's why I know how important it is to bring a more mindful approach to it.

There are as many attitudes toward money as there are people. What I consider a lot of money may seem derisory to you, and vice versa. Neither of us is necessarily wrong. As with so many beliefs, our views about money are so ingrained that we don't even realize we have them. And, as with most beliefs, I reckon it makes sense to challenge them, and check they're useful, helpful and align with our values, to ensure we're living the life we want, not the one others told us we should.

The key is to figure out what you think about money, and not be influenced by parents, friends or prevailing culture. Just because your parents counted every penny or spent thousands on wine, or your friend makes it clear that a monthly £200 food spend is shocking (even though you know someone else who spends that on a single lunch), it doesn't mean you have to agree.

Money myths

Unhelpful money beliefs and behaviours are commonly known in coaching as "money mindset blocks". These usually refer to personal beliefs about money, which can cause you to sabotage your own relationship with work, finances and earning.

Some common "blocks" include:

- Your work is more noble if you're not well-paid
- Doing work you love can't pay the bills
- Only "sensible jobs" are well-paid (e.g. lawyer, banker, doctor...)
- Asking for more money is daring
- You don't deserve (and shouldn't want) to be paid for doing work you enjoy
- You shouldn't spend money on yourself
- The only sensible thing to do with money is to save it
- Budgeting is boring and the opposite of spontaneity
- Enjoying money is frivolous
- Talking about money is rude

- Seeking money makes you "flash" and lacks class
- All rich people are arrogant snobs
- All the best people are humble and live frugally
- The best things in life are always free

I could go on. The central idea is to realize that, just like with many other thoughts you may have, these beliefs are not necessarily true, correct or helpful. Part of rewiring our brains for success includes rooting out unhelpful beliefs and reframing them, so we can live a life that feels good.

FINANCIAL WELLBEING

The term "financial wellbeing" has become a bit of a psychological buzzword in recent years. It's well overdue, I think, when money can otherwise become such a source of stress.

Financial services provider Aegon defines financial wellbeing as: "How people feel about the control they have over their financial future – and their relationship with money. It's about focusing on the things that make their life enjoyable and meaningful."[1]

A 2020 report from the UK National Forum for Health and Wellbeing at Work found that, unsurprisingly, a lack of financial wellbeing had the potential to cause "financial and mental trauma".[2]

Over the past few years, as a business owner in pursuit of my own definition of financial wellbeing, I have had to confront my "money blocks" regularly. I started out believing that only certain jobs deserved to be paid well, that my skills were not worth paying for, and that choosing to start my own business meant that I would inevitably make less than I would if I had stayed in my 9-to-5 job. Because my salary as a full-time staff journalist, despite my degrees and experience, had peaked at £30,000, I came to believe that my work and *therefore my value as a human*, was probably only worth about that, too.

I used to think that caring about money was the most boring thing *ever*. I also thought being "rich" and "successful" meant being rude and aloof, dripping with Hermès, flying to St Tropez because you felt like it, and always being just a little bit drunk and unhappy. I somehow also thought it meant never needing to look at your bank balance, cavorting around in a power suit in a glass office, or lounging in a designer sarong on a massive yacht by a Greek island.

None of these things are true. Don't get me wrong, I love a Greek island as much as the next girl (more, probably), but I now know that making your own money can mean whatever the heck you want it to.

And, incidentally, I make much more now than I ever did when I worked in my 9-to-5, so *that* myth about my "worth" didn't turn out to be true either *hair toss*.

Millionaire, don't care

I now know that as many people make millions at home in yoga pants and unwashed hair as they do in suits in shiny offices, and both are fine, if that's what you want. You can choose what you spend your money on. You can make ethical and powerful choices if you want to. Having more money doesn't make you a better or worse person, and what you spend your money on doesn't necessarily make you more noble, or vice versa. The idea that you can detach your beliefs around money and instead choose whatever you want to believe about it, and therefore your ability to get it, is pretty damn freeing.

Yes, all of us need a certain amount to survive, and there are certainly more worthwhile causes to invest in or donate to than others. And of course, I am absolutely not suggesting that all we need to do to get more money is change our mindset or beliefs around it. But I do believe that, provided we have enough to live on in the first place, trying to improve our thoughts around money and taking a more mindful approach to what we *do* have, can reap huge benefits.

As the famous 2012 poll by the Marist Institute for Public Opinion showed, our happiness generally increases as our income rises above $50,000 (£36,000), but a study from Princeton University showed that this happiness levels off after about $75,000 (£54,000). Beyond that, the study found, people continued to rate their lives as more satisfying, but they didn't seem to experience any more happiness on a day-to-day basis.[3] Don't get me wrong, £36,000–£54,000 sounds pretty good to me... but it's a lot less than some might expect would equal blissful happiness.

Not to mention, what "happiness" actually looks like is totally yours to decide, and all the money in the world won't help you if you have no budget, no goals and no gratitude for what you *do* have. As Elizabeth Dunn, associate professor of psychology at the University of British Columbia and author of *Happy Money: The Science of Smarter Spending*, told *Time* magazine: "It turns out, what you do with your money seems to matter as much to your happiness as how much you make."[4]

The more I learn about money – the more encouraged, grateful and intentional I am about it – the more it feels like I have, and the more easily it seems to come to me via new work opportunities. Not only that, but the more I shift my beliefs about money, and see it as a positive thing rather that something to be afraid of, the more hopeful I am that mindful people making good money can save the world through their responsible, kind choices.

But let's climb down a rung or two from those lofty goals for a second. How, in practice, can we unpick our own beliefs about money, and how can we be more mindful about it for better results, on a day-to-day level? Because I am far from a financial guru, I figured it would make sense to ask some actual money experts about this.

Spend according to your values

First, I spoke to Chelsea Garcia, a financial coach and author of the book *S.A.V.E. Yourself: Develop the Financial Fitness to Spend in Alignment with your Values, not Ego*.[5] I asked her what that means, and how it helps us to spend and live more mindfully. She told me:

"We often feel as though we have two voices in us. The one that encourages us to act from our highest and best self, our values; and the one that is like, 'Live for now, you only live once!' – your ego.

"So many of us are in financial trouble because the ego speaks first and loudest. It's always going to be there. But we want to quiet it down, and to raise the volume of our values. I know people can resist being mindful about money because it seems so fun to be mind*less* about it. But that's not sustainable.

"We have to ask, what does mindful spending look like? The answer begins with meditation. Because meditating will help you define success for yourself. It doesn't mean that you can't have nice things. It just means that you know for yourself what's enough.

"When I start helping people, I ask them: 'What do you think your values are?' And they say, for example: 'Spending time with family.' But when we look at their receipts, it's all online shopping, not family stuff. So the way they're spending their money is inconsistent with what's important to them. And then they're upset because they think they don't have enough money.

"And I say, 'No, it's just that you're spending your money *incorrectly*, compared to what will actually make you happy."[6]

Define your "enough"

Chelsea advises us to "Start with meditation… that gets you in touch with your own vision for what success looks like, separate from the one we are taught", and ask yourself:

- What's "enough money" for you?
- What would be enough clothes/a big enough house/ enough eating out/travel for you?
- What are your values, and how can you make your spending reflect them?

Then, create a plan to spend your money from that place. Every day, you can make choices about how you spend your money, in alignment with your values (what you stand for):

- Imagine that your money is a pie, equal to 100%.
- Decide what's important to you, and allocate a percentage of the pie to each.
- Then take those percentages and apply them to your current income.

According to Chelsea, that's what spending your money according to your values looks like.

Obviously, she says, sometimes we have to be realistic. "We would all love to live in a castle that costs $5 a month to rent, and have no bills. But if you're spending proportionally more on housing [than you thought], maybe it means that where you live is more important to you than you realized."

Chelsea told me how having a plan can also remove the guilt and shame you might normally have about spending. She said: "I remember I had one client who loved baseball and always felt guilty for spending money on it. But she realized it was important to her, and so allocated money to it every month. Next time she went to a Dodger game, she got a hot dog and a pointy foam finger. And she told me: 'The best part was that I didn't feel the guilt that I normally do. I had set this money aside to spend, whereas before, I would have told myself that these hot dogs are way too expensive, and been like, who needs a stupid foam finger?' But with her new system, she was able to fully be present and enjoy the moment. And her life felt richer."

Money is power

But of course, money isn't just about being able to enjoy ourselves. It can also be a powerful tool in helping us to feel confident and in control, make decisions that benefit us, and help us show up as the powerful woman we want to be.

That's why I also spoke to Rebecca Freeman, founder of Lagom Finance (*lagom* means "not too much, not too little, just right", in Swedish – isn't that great?). She offers accountancy services for female-led businesses who want control, clarity and peace of mind over their finances. *Yes, please.*

I asked her how to start to become more mindful about managing our business money and our mindset.[7]

The CEO mindset

She said: "Even if you've got a 'side hustle', I'd encourage you to think of yourself as the CEO of your company, rather than saying: 'Oh, it's this little thing I do a couple of nights a week.' That isn't going to do you any favours. I would say, plan for it to be really successful from day one. Even if you don't want to be CEO of a big company, just knowing that you're doing it for good reasons, such as supporting your children or having enough to buy your dream house, puts you in a different frame of mind."

Charging your worth

"Women so often don't charge what they're worth. This especially happens with side hustles. Women think, 'I'm doing this on the side, so I can just charge, like, £10 an hour.' But by doing that, you're saying your work is only *worth* that amount per hour, which isn't the case. Ultimately, you end up resenting your clients because you haven't been paid enough for the time. So setting your prices at what you need to earn, and valuing your experience and time, is so important. It's probably taken me the last five years to realize that!"

(I would add a caveat here: "charging your worth" doesn't mean charging what you are worth as a human, or equating your work with your worth. No price equals that! It's just about valuing your skills and time, and charging what feels good and makes it worth your while. It's about doing your research and charging the market rate, rather than undercutting yourself.)

Reframe your money story

Rebecca also advises women to become more aware of their attitude toward money, and stop telling themselves they're "bad with it". She told me: "Everyone's money story is different. What I think is being 'great with money' might be completely different to you. I think a lot of guilt comes from women feeling they're 'not good with money'. But not everyone is a numbers person. I'm not – I can't do crazy calculations in my head like Russell Crowe in *A Beautiful Mind*."[8]

Rebecca advises the following:

• Stop saying you're "bad with money", or "not a numbers person".

- Instead, reframe it as something like: "I'm working on being confident with money." This, she says, will change your mindset with a view to creating real-life change.
- Don't expect change overnight. Commit to changing or saving one thing per month, and see the changes add up slowly but surely.

Make a money date with yourself

Happily, Rebecca also advises everyone to make a regular "money date" with ourselves, so we make staying aware of it a pleasurable thing.

- Make a money date with yourself in your calendar, either weekly or monthly.
- Make it fun. Get a good bottle of wine or cheese, for example!
- Take half an hour to an hour to review where you're at with your finances.
- Don't bury your head in the sand. Get all your accounts together, and really look at what you can afford, and plan ahead.

She explains: "When you're busy running your business every day, you don't get that space to sit down and think about the next 12 months. But this way, you can make it fun rather than fearful."

More money, cheese and wine, and a life that feels mentally and literally richer? Sounds like a plan to me. And as Rebecca told me: "It all starts with awareness."

Examples of reframing unhelpful money beliefs	
Doing work you love can't possibly pay the bills. Only "sensible jobs" are well-paid.	A lot of people do work they love that pays the bills, such as actors, artists, writers, chefs, sports stars... Why not me?
Asking for money for something I enjoy doing is daring or shocking.	Asking to be paid for my skills and time is not shocking. I wouldn't ask a trained hairdresser or mechanic to cut my hair or service my car for free.
I must burn myself out and work ridiculously hard to be worthy of payment.	Burning myself out will mean I can't serve my clients, and helps no-one. The healthier I am, the better my work is too.

MEDITATION TOOL

Visualization for success

Imagine yourself in five to ten years, living and breathing your definition of success. What do you see? What are you doing? Where are you? What can you hear, touch, taste, smell? Who is with you (or absent)? What do you do with your days? How have you achieved this success?

Notice any feelings, sensations or thoughts that make themselves known as you watch. How do the sensations change, if at all?

If you get distracted, just notice that and bring your attention back when you can.

15

Meditation for Activism and Actual Change

(or, Mindfulness in the Real World)

"We can't meditate away the injustice, the oppression, the pain, the suffering... but we can have some measure of perspective... and balance. So we can respond with clarity and kindness. Our meditation practice is very important. We can't only look inside. We have to be willing to see what's in front of us."

Sebene Selassie, meditation teacher, author and speaker

Perhaps inevitably, mindfulness has been subject to backlash in recent years – some of it rightfully. The main criticism I've seen is from Ronald Purser, who wrote a book called *McMindfulness*. The term "McMindfulness" was coined by Miles Neale, a Buddhist teacher and psychotherapist, to describe "spiritual practices that provide immediate nutrition but not long-term sustenance".[1]

Building on this idea, Purser has lampooned the popularization of mindfulness, and criticized it for being marketed as a "magic panacea", when in fact it is, he says, "nothing more than basic concentration training" that is "void of a moral compass", which has been "commodified and oversold", and fails to face up to the real problems of the modern world. He writes:

> "I am sceptical. Anything that offers success in our unjust society without trying to change it is not revolutionary – it just helps people cope. However, it could also be making things worse. Instead of encouraging radical action, it says the causes of suffering are disproportionately inside us, not in the political and economic frameworks that shape how we live."[2]

As I've said already, the usual definition of mindfulness is "Paying attention, in the present moment, on purpose, without judgement." But as I've also said, if you take only one thing away from this book, it should be that "paying attention", or "concentration", as Purser calls it, *should not be the only aim.* While there is some relief in gaining perspective on our thoughts, simply *being aware* of things won't fix them. We need compassion for that.

Get fixed quick

But admittedly, most of us do come to meditation because we are seeking relief from our own anxiety, overwhelm or depression. It's understandable, at least at first, that we might become blind to anything except easing our pain. This is like using meditation the way we might pop a painkiller for a headache. It works fine, at first. But once the headache recedes, we might then want to look at why we get headaches in the first place.

(I'm all for medication, by the way. Painkillers, anti-depressants, all good. As long as they're taken with awareness, used with caution, and used in conjunction with other mental and physical health improvements, too.)

But many people continue to use meditation to treat the symptoms without taking the time to look at their cause.

- Employer asking you to do three jobs? Meditate away your stress and keep going!
- Unable to access good healthcare? Just learn to mindfully reduce pain with this helpful online mindfulness-based stress reduction (MBSR) course!
- Getting headaches because you spend your whole life in front of a screen? Fix it by closing your eyes for five minutes and noticing how you feel!

Anxious AF because of climate change? Terrified by systemic racism, misogyny, conspiracy theorists and the post-fact world? Feel like a total failure every time you scroll through Instagram? Simple! Just do some mindful breathing exercises and name five things you can see, touch, smell, hear or taste! Breathe! The problem is inside your head! Fix that, problem solved!

This is obviously sarcasm. Despite my tone, in some ways, this isn't *all bad*. I obviously believe meditation *can* and *does* offer relief for all of these things. But the whitewashing and commodification of mindfulness – the way it has been packaged up into neat eight-week programmes that fit into corporate budgets for burned-out employees – and is associated with super-expensive studios and yoga mats that cost half a month's rent – mean that it's increasingly easy for it to make fools of us all. We're stressed out by corporate society, but then corporate society turns around to sell us the solution. I agree, it stinks.

McMindfulness

This so-called "McMindfulness" strips meditation of its ethics, and sells it back to us at inflated prices with all the ease and nutritional emptiness of a Happy Meal®. We get "calming" Buddha statues in gardens, bathrooms, hairdressing salons and restaurants. We get "mindful" tea, "mindful" sleep spray, "mindful" food kits, "mindful" colouring books, and are told that meditation will solve all our problems (even the truly severe ones).

We are told that the aim is to get so relaxed that we no longer care that we have to work 80 hours a week, and that the world is burning. And if we still feel terrible, or we can't afford or fit into the correct yoga pants to do it in, then we're made to feel as though we're doing it wrong. It's the ultimate in gaslighting.

A quote often attributed to the philosopher Jiddu Krishnamurti (but some dispute this) said, "It is no measure of health to be well-adjusted to a profoundly sick society."[3] On this idea, Purser and I appear to agree. Meditation should *not* be used purely as a self-help to optimize your brain for better output, or to become more inward-looking only, or as a sticking plaster for burnout or an unsustainable lifestyle.

Genuine meditation is not just an app on your phone, a habit to "tick off" on your Optimised Morning Routine™ or another trophy to place on your desk without any awareness of the history or wider societal implications. To see it in this way, or to think that it is to be mainly used for this purpose, is to dismiss 95% of its origins and content, and to do it a massive disservice.

Modern mindfulness

But here's where Mr McMindfulness and I part ways. As far as I can see, Purser's reading of modern mindfulness is utterly cynical. He has cherry-picked a few examples of ways in which the practice has been commodified and taught without enough respect for ethics, and decided that this is the only way that mindfulness exists now.

He has taken a few random quotes from mindfulness scientist Jon Kabat-Zinn, and suggested that "awareness" and "paying attention" are the entire endgame. But the phrase "happiness is an inside job" doesn't mean that people who meditate should not, cannot – or are never encouraged to – be aware of what's on the outside.

Purser takes issue with the marketing of mindfulness, which he says, is "excised" of its Buddhism in an "insulting" way, and offers "Buddhist meditation without the Buddhism".[4] But he appears to take the definition of "paying attention without judgement" at face value, and criticizes all modern mindfulness. He seems to suggest that the modern selling of secular "awareness without *judgement*" means "not giving a shit about anything or anyone except yourself", and purely using meditation for selfish aims.

Believe me, if Ron Purser ever reads this and feels I've completely misunderstood his message, then I'll be more than happy to discuss it further.

But, as far as I can tell, his critique is a damaging misreading of the intentions of most sincere, modern meditation – even Westernized meditation packaged up for non-Buddhists. It is my firm view that you don't have to be a Buddhist, or spiritual, to meditate properly.

I do believe, however, that as meditators, we have a responsibility to be aware that it's *not* purely about attention training, or who becomes the most productive, or who clocks up the most minutes on their smartphone app, or who becomes the "best meditator". It's also about *ethics*, and becoming more aware and compassionate in general. The two are not mutually exclusive. Done correctly, meditation not only helps us ease our own suffering, but opens us up to that of others even more intensely, so that we are not merely aware of it, but increasingly likely to *do* something about it.

Studies bear this out. In 2013, researchers at the Max Planck Institute in Germany taught volunteers a version of loving-kindness (or compassion) meditation. They then showed the volunteers images of people suffering, and found that after just eight hours of practice, the volunteers' responses changed from simple empathy (feeling their pain too), to feeling *love* – of the kind usually felt by parents for children – toward those who were suffering, when compared to volunteers who hadn't been taught loving-kindness.[5] Another study, in 2013, found people who had practised loving-kindness were twice as likely to give up their seat for someone who needed it, compared to people who didn't practise.[6]

All of this goes to say that, yes, the happiness and productivity that Purser takes such issue with are lovely by-products of meditation. But good meditation will *also* likely make you give less of a crap about job titles and toxic workplace culture, and teach you to care more about the impact your company might be having on society at large.

Meditation is absolutely *not* about selfish goals, easing our pain without ever caring about anyone else's, or numbing us to an increasingly overwhelming and troubling society. It's the opposite. It can make us *more* conscious and compassionate, not the "optimized" self-obsessed worker bees that Purser seems to think we all aspire to be.

Modern meditation can build compassion

If, through "paying attention", we see our own feelings of sadness, exhaustion, overwhelm, inadequacy and pain, then we will be less able to turn a blind eye when we see it in other people. It is by first focusing on the self, that we are better able to help others.

The word "compassion" literally comes from the Latin, "compatī" meaning "suffer *with*". As far as I'm aware, we as humans haven't yet found a reliable way to feel others' pain physically. All we can do is get very still and very aware and compassionate to our own pain, and use that to build our empathy toward others.

In fact, in their book *The Science of Meditation*, meditation researchers Richard J. Davidson and Daniel Goleman hammer home the importance of ethics, and readily admit, "Quite a lot has been left behind as the world's rich contemplative traditions morphed into user-friendly forms..." They add, "Historically, meditation was not meant to improve our health, relax us, or enhance work success... Such benefits were incidental, unnoted side-effects." Instead, they say that "deep" meditation is "just one part of a range of means helping to increase self-awareness... and ultimately, to achieve a lasting transformation of being." They then list "an ethical stance, altruistic intention, community, and a supportive culture" as some of the other necessary parts."[7]

I could not agree more.

Learn about the origins of meditation

It's easy for the goals of modern meditation to be misconstrued. Maybe unsurprisingly, I have personally been publicly accused of appropriation, and of perpetuating mindfulness as a "whitewashed" Western idea, and being disrespectful in how I talk about it. And I get why, even if I don't agree.

Many people may well believe that meditation *should* remain a spiritual practice delivered by monks or nuns who have spent years in silent retreats. Fair enough. If that's what you're looking for, I genuinely hope you find it. There is so much wisdom there, I don't disagree completely. In fact, all the Western teachers of mindfulness and meditation – from Jon Kabat-Zinn to Sharon Salzberg, to Jack Kornfield to Joseph Goldstein, and more – have spent serious time in India, Myanmar, Vietnam and Thailand, before coming back to the West to spread the word. Some of the most popular teachers *are* monks or nuns – such as Thich Nhat Hanh or

Pema Chödrön – and I have enormous respect for them. How could I not?

But just because these practices originated in the East, doesn't mean they can't apply in the West. I truly believe that no-one is the gatekeeper of meditation, and that no-one "owns" it. I only ever see myself as passing on the tools of meditation as I keep learning, acting as a conduit for teachings that began centuries ago. As long as you're respectful, educate yourself about the difference between appreciation and appropriation, and have some knowledge of its origins and history, then I firmly believe you can meditate sincerely without being a Buddhist, or even being that spiritual. As the Dalai Lama, arguably the world's most famous Buddhist, says, "Know the rules... so you can break them effectively."

WHITEWASHING

There is a more sinister but important point to be made here about white people "appropriating" things, and taking only the pretty parts of someone else's culture and making them "palatable", while forgetting the real roots and meaning, which is always offensive and wrong. I actually believe that skinny white women have become associated with yoga and meditation in the West exactly *because* our culture celebrates them to the expense of all other types of bodies, so naturally these women appear more *visible* than others. They absolutely shouldn't, but they do. And I reckon the *reason* so many white people found yoga and meditation *in the first place* is because the Western dominant culture made them so damn miserable, they were – justifiably – looking for an exit. It's just a tragic shame that in doing so, these white proponents have unwittingly perpetuated so many of the harmful, toxic practices they were trying to escape.

As the yoga teacher, woman of colour, body positivity advocate and writer Jessamyn Stanley (at the phenomenally successful Instagram account @mynameisjessamyn) writes about yoga: "As much as social media has given me, it shouldn't be the only source of inspiration for people who don't fit the typical yoga mold... All yoga bodies deserve to be represented... not just those that are slender, female, and white."[8]

I feel the exact same way about meditation.

This is not to excuse the harmful appropriation and whitewashing that we so often see, but as a white woman trying to educate myself, I see it as my responsibility to be aware of these issues, and to work to educate other white people who might need it, too. It's not up to anyone else to do it for us.

Mindfulness is accessible to all

And yet, I also believe in making meditation more accessible, whether that's using the word "badass" in my brand name, or swearing gently on a guided track. In fact, I was drawn to Buddhism precisely because others have gone before me to make it more accessible. As I've mentioned before, when I first discovered my Buddhist meditation teacher's book *The Buddha Walks Into a Bar* and saw the phrase, "No teacher said the best way to create inner change is to be a prick to yourself",[9] and I discovered Liza Kindred's Instagram account "Eff This! Meditation (@effthismeditation)", I knew I'd found my people.

Contrary to popular belief, you do *not* have to have a collection of crystals, incense, sage or eye-wateringly expensive yoga pants and a meditation cushion to meditate. You *can*. Your butt will look great and your house will smell lovely. But you don't *have* to. I mean no harm to people who enjoy all those things, but they can so easily come off as smug, woo, weird or flat-out unattainable for the rest of us who just want to feel less stressed on a Tuesday night.

At its core, meditation is a great leveller. At its most basic and raw, it's free (just use your breath and body), portable, discreet and available to anyone with any kind of body.

As long as you can breathe or feel in some way, and you're taught with awareness, compassion and in a trauma-informed way, meditation is open to you, regardless of race, income, size, ability, sexuality, background, job, religion or surroundings. As it should be.

From whitewashing to activism

But it's not enough to make meditation less whitewashed and more accessible. To help us become better humans, we must also use our increased awareness and compassion to improve society.

Being aware, angry and outspoken about injustices – and becoming aware of our privilege and how that colours how we see the world – is not incompatible with mindfulness. We can be mindful, rational and calm – *as well as* mad as hell. Sam Harris, neuroscientist, philosopher, author, podcaster and founder of the meditation app Wake Up,[10] has recently spoken about how that anger, activism and mindfulness are not mutually exclusive. In an interview with Dan Harris (no relation) on the 10% Happier podcast, Sam said:

> *"[I'm] very active on Twitter... and there are people who see that and think: 'Hey, you could use your own meditation app! What the hell are you doing? Who are you to teach [people] to meditate if you're so caught up by politics?' But I think that emotions like outrage, and anger, and fear, are salient signals that are worth paying attention to."* [11]

He explains that just because we are angry, it doesn't mean we stay angry forever. It also doesn't mean we cannot be angry on one hand, and be rational and focused on the other, drawing light to injustice and working on combatting the source of our anger. Emotions are not binary.

And he is also clear that we do not meditate to become calm to the point that we never have any emotions or any inclination to speak up for what we believe in. He says:

> *"It's not that I never get bent out of shape... [but] to be silent, as the arsonist is busily lighting a fire to everything*

you care about, that is a failure to understand what the
[aim is] to maintain human wellbeing."[12]

Be open to suffering, without being poisoned

The Vietnamese Buddhist monk and spiritual leader Thich Nhat Hanh has spent almost an entire lifetime showing how Buddhist principles can make us better activists, if used well. He has said: "Our own life has to be the message," and in his seminal book *Peace Is Every Step* he wrote: "When you begin to see that your enemy is suffering, that is the beginning of insight."[13] In another of his books *Anger: Wisdom for Cooling the Flames* he wrote: "The fact is that when you make the other suffer, he will try to find relief by making you suffer more. The result is an escalation of suffering on both sides."[14]

As today's world seems ever-more polarized, and bitter debates still rage over topics such as Black Lives Matter, LGBTQIA rights, Brexit, divided politics, COVID, violence against women and beyond, maintaining this level of compassion has never been more challenging or needed.

We all have a responsibility to stand up for what we think is right, while also listening to others with different lived experiences – shutting up and listening when appropriate, and understanding how our privilege and experience has informed the way we think. We can stand by our view of the world, at the same time as being open to others' views. We can use mindfulness to gain insight and perspective outside of our own echo chamber. We can use it to de-escalate conflict, and aim to come to a resolution or change, without totally sacrificing our values. It's not easy, but it's a good aim to have.

As Tim Desmond, psychotherapist, student of Thich Nhat Hanh, and author of *How To Stay Human in A F*cked Up World*, writes, "It's possible to pay attention and care about the suffering in the world without letting it poison us."[15] And when I asked him onto my podcast to explain, he told me that as a poor child of a single alcoholic mother from a rough part of Boston, by the time he got to college on a sports scholarship, he was "pretty lonely and angry".[16]

When he discovered the work of Thich Nhat Hanh, Tim realized that "mindfulness and compassion" was what was missing from his life. The more he learned, the more he became involved with the monk's work, and with political grassroots organizing. And he saw how the compassion and stability he had been developing in himself could be applied to protest movements. He told me:

> "[From] mindfulness, I learned that it's possible to be happy, and relate to life in such a way that you're happy to be alive. And that capacity to be happy to be alive is an energy that helps you to be more of service to others. What the fuck else would I want to do? What's the use of a human life if it's not to benefit yourself and others? I want to be of service to the world. I want my life to matter."[17]

He explained that, rather than using mindfulness as a way to *escape from* our problems, we can instead ask ourselves the following questions and "let that be our fuel":

- How do I apply these teachings to something I feel alive for?
- What motivates me?
- Why am I here?
- Why do I care about meditation?
- Why do I care about mindfulness?
- Why do I care about any self-development?

Similarly, as meditation teacher Sebene Selassie says, our aim with meditation should not be to "meditate away the injustice, the oppression, the pain, the suffering", but instead use it as an insightful tool for "perspective and grounding, and balance", so we can "respond with clarity and kindness" and "see what's in front of us".[18]

When the tragedies with Breonna Taylor and George Floyd – and so many others – happened in 2020, the penny *finally* dropped for many white people that we still have so much more to learn about the trauma and racism still happening in the US, UK and beyond.

Even those of us who had attempted to learn about racism previously were confronted with the reality that posting a black square on Instagram was *not helpful.* Despite what we had always been taught, articulating our views was not, in this case, helpful or right.

Instead, what we needed to do – and must continue to do – is to be quiet. We must listen carefully, and learn from the incredible educators who take their precious time to educate us. We must educate ourselves too, donate where we can, attend marches and raise awareness, listen to others' lived experiences, and speak out against racism or sexism and other injustices, one comment at a time.

It turns out that mindfulness and meditation are potent tools to help us do just that. When we increase our ability to listen, learn, change our own behaviour and patterns, and apply compassion and understanding to our own suffering, we also increase our ability to do exactly that toward others.

Ultimately, meditation and mindfulness are tools that help us rewire our brain for more awareness and compassion, so it makes sense that they help us open our eyes to the suffering of others, and become more aware of our privilege, and our responsibility to the world.

To ignore that aspect of the practice, and to use it purely as a way of making yourself feel calmer after a long day in the office, is to see only one tiny part of it. Meditation must be seen as part of a wider body of ethics. Taking the "awareness" and "focus" elements of it and leaving the rest is an incomplete reading of the practice itself. Meditation isn't magic, but it is a bit of a real-life superpower – not only enabling us to help ourselves, but also making us more willing and equipped to help others, too.

MEDITATION TOOL

Loving-kindness toward others

In a seated meditation position, close your eyes, if you choose, and bring your attention to any areas of your body that feel good. Breathe normally.

Hold an image of yourself in your mind, and repeat: "May I be safe, may I be happy, may I be healthy, may I feel good in my body." Repeat at a speed that feels natural. Change or add to the phrases if you like, to ensure they really resonate with you. Repeat. Notice how you feel, without judgement.

Then bring someone you love to mind. Repeat the phrases to them: "May *you* be safe, may *you* be happy," etc. Repeat.

Then bring someone neutral to mind, who you don't really know. It might be a delivery driver, or a supermarket worker. Repeat the phrases toward them.

Then bring someone to mind who you struggle with. Maybe an old colleague, a friend who hurt you. Start with someone easy, and work up. Repeat the phrases to them, too. Remember that, even though they hurt you, they're probably hurting; they are human, just like you.

Repeat.

MEDITATION TOOL

Sitting with discomfort

Once seated in meditation, breathe in for a count of three, and breathe out for four. Repeat.

With each exhale, allow your muscles to relax, and melt down into your seat, while keeping your spine straight and alert.

Close your eyes if you like. Know that you're safe, solid and grounded where you are, and you can always stop if you choose.

Now imagine a situation that makes you slightly uncomfortable, or someone saying something you really don't agree with. What physical reactions come up immediately? Do you feel tense, hot, resistant, angry?

Notice the sensations, and then try to relax around them, rather than resisting. Breathe.

What changes do you notice? Can you question your original reaction? Might there be a calmer, more helpful, or kinder way to respond?

The End of the Beginning

This is not an end point. It's just the beginning.

Sometimes it feels as though the secret to life is realizing that, basically, none of us have our shit together, at least not all of the time.

My writing a book like this might make it look like I have my shit together, and that there's nothing more to add or learn. Nope. It's the opposite. "Do this, and just like me, you will be cured!" is exactly what I'm *not* trying to say.

Instead, I reckon that we're all just making it up as we go along, figuring out what works for us, leaving what doesn't, and – crucially – learning to be genuinely happy with that. And being on your own side is a bloody good place to start. I hope this book helps with that.

As for me, I have had the privilege of learning from some incredible teachers along the way, and it's in their wonderful company, with words of wisdom from four excellent women, that I leave you.

"Meditation is the key to knowing yourself."

Pema Chödrön, Buddhist nun

"You yourself, as much as anybody in the entire universe, deserve your love and affection."

Sharon Salzberg, meditation teacher

"Instructions for living a life: pay attention. Be astonished. Tell about it."
"Tell me, what is it you plan to do with your one wild and precious life?"

Mary Oliver, poet and writer

"Life feels so much more playful when your sense of identity isn't pinned to accomplishment. You can be an ambitious person, without feeling like the outcome means something about you. You can make things happen in a playful way when you don't pin the outcome to your sense of self-worth. Everything in your life could crumble down around you right now... and you'd still be enough."

Adreanna Limbach, meditation teacher

If you remember only these five points from this entire book... I reckon that will be enough, too.

Acknowledgements

Thanks must first go to my teachers, all of whom have shared their incredible, peaceful, measured and immense wisdom with me, and continue to do so.

Thanks especially to Lodro Rinzler and Adreanna Limbach (and everyone I have met through them) and Marie Johansson at the Oxford Mindfulness Centre for their wisdom, humour, patience and guidance.

Thanks also to these teachers and writers – some of whom I've spoken with and met in person, but most I have not and likely never will. Most of you don't know me, but you have helped me and my work more than you will ever know (in no particular order!): Brené Brown, Pema Chödrön, Glennon Doyle, Carol S. Dweck, Anushka Fernandopulle, Joseph Goldstein, Daniel Goleman and Richard J. Davidson, Thich Nhat Hanh, JoAnna Hardy, Liza Kindred, Dan Harris, Jon Kabat-Zinn, Cory Muscara, Andy Puddicombe, Sharon Salzberg, Sebene Selassie, David A. Treleaven, Jeff Warren and Light Watkins.

To my badass one-to-one clients, who never stop amazing me with their resilience, self-awareness, courage, humour and commitment, and who give me a reason to keep doing this work, even when I'm convinced no-one cares and it's a waste of time. Thank you.

To all of my wonderful podcast guests, I thank you for sharing your boundless knowledge and enthusiasm and love for life with me, as well as your appreciation for chocolate, sourdough bread, reality TV… and deep conversations about being human.

To my friends, who kept me going via WhatsApp, Zoom and Instagram across oceans and lockdowns, and who offered to read and buy this book long before it was even written, and who kept their promise even *after* it was done – you are the best badasses I know.

To my business coaches, including Jereshia Hawk and Tyler J. McCall, for showing me what is possible in the world of online business, and enabling me to make this my career.

To Beth, my lovely editor, who asked if I'd like to write a book, and then braced herself for perhaps the biggest word-cutting job of her life once she realized quite how much I *did* want to write one. Thank you for stewarding my project with humour and ease, and for emailing me in the first place. You're the reason this actually exists.

To Powell's Books in Portland, Oregon, for inspiring me. To Valletta, Malta and to Álora Yurts and Mijas Pueblo in Spain, for reminding me that sunshine, hope and blue sky is out there, even if I can't always see it from here.

To my parents and family, who are always there for me, no matter what, even when they have no idea what the actual heck I'm doing or why.

To my "parents in not-law" (my partner's parents) for cheering me on, for remembering when my writing deadlines were, and for generally being more supportive thay anyone could expect.

ACKNOWLEDGEMENTS

And to Oli, who already knows how much he helped me write this book, mainly just by being there, by supporting and challenging my ideas, reminding me to close my laptop, rest and eat properly every now and again, for believing in and loving me when I'm struggling to believe in or love myself, and for being the best partner – in all senses of the word – that I could ever wish for. Love you.

Endnotes

Part One: The Basics

1. Why Should I Meditate?

1. D. Harris, J. Warren with C. Adler, *Meditation For Fidgety Skeptics: A 10% Happier How-To Book*, Yellow Kite, 2018.

2. T. Chodron, *Don't Believe Everything You Think: Living with Wisdom and Compassion*, Snow Lion, 2013.

3. D. Goleman and R. Davidson, *The Science of Meditation: How to Change Your Brain, Mind and Body*, Penguin, 2017.

4. *Ibid.* p. 250.

5. *Ibid.* p. 251.

2. Is Meditation Really for Me?

1. S. Salzberg, *Real Happiness: The Power of Meditation: A 28-Day Program*, Highbridge Co., 2011.

2. H. Thompson and L. Kindred, "Ep #11: Mindful Tech, Self-Love, and Meditation For Your Real, Actual Life", June 29, 2019. In *The Breathe Like A Badass Podcast*, Podcast, MP3 audio, www.breathelikeabadass.com/podcast

3. A How-to Guide to Beginners' Meditation

1. D. Harris and J. Biewen, "Ep #333: The Self-Interested Case for Examining Your Biases | John Biewen", 2020. In *Ten Percent Happier with Dan Harris*, by ABC Audio. Podcast. https://www.tenpercent.com/podcast-episode/john-biewen-333

2. C. Muscara, @corymuscara, May 10, 2020. Instagram. https://www.instagram.com/p/CAArmtOnhtP

3. G. Doyle, *Untamed: Stop Pleasing, Start Living*, Ebury Digital, 2020.

4. N. Antoinette, 2021. In *Real Talk Radio Podcast*, Podcast, https://realtalkradiopodcast.com

5. S. Selassie, "Getting Out of Your Head: Mindfulness is a Misnomer", Sebene Selassie Blog, 2021. https://www.sebeneselassie.com/blog/getting-out-of-your-head-mindfulness-is-a-misnomer

6. Headspace Inc., *Headspace: Meditation & Sleep*, Headspace Inc., 2021.

7. 10% Happier Inc., *Ten Percent Happier Meditation*, 10% Happier Inc., 2021.

8. M. Maehlum, *Momentum Habit Tracker – Routines, Goals & Rituals*, Momentum.cc, 2015.

9. Apalon App, *Productive – Habit Tracker*, IAC Search & Media Technologies Limited, 2014–2021.

10. G. Chapman, *The Five Love Languages: The Secret to Love That Lasts*, Moody Press, 2009.

11. The 5 Love Languages® Quiz for Singles, Northfield Publishing, Grooters Productions, Moody Publishers, 2021. https://www.5lovelanguages.com/quizzes/singles-quiz/

12. S. Beckett, *Worstward Ho*, Grove Pr, 1984.

Part Two: Meditation in Practice

4. Meditation for Self-Compassion

1. R. Knight, "Eight in 10 young adults feel they are not good enough, poll claims", *Independent*, 2019. https://www.independent.co.uk/news/uk/home-news/millennials-mental-health-love-young-adults-social-media-poll-alpro-a9181296.html

2. A. Limbach, *Tea and Cake with Demons: A Buddhist Guide to Feeling Worthy*, Sounds True, 2019.

3. H. Thompson and A. Limbach, "Ep #13: Adreanna Limbach: How To Make Peace With Your Demons & Finally Feel Good Enough (with Buddhism, Tea, & Cake)", August 12, 2019. In *The Breathe Like A Badass Podcast*, Podcast, MP3 audio, breathelikeabadass.com/podcast

4. C. Caldwell, "In a society that profits from your self-doubt, liking yourself is a rebellious act", artwork, 2015. https://www.rebelliousact.org

5. K. Neff, *Self-Compassion: Stop Beating Yourself Up and Leave Insecurity Behind*, Hodder & Stoughton, 2011, p. 85.

6. A. Kendrick, "Oh God. I just realized I'm stuck with me my whole life.", Tweet, May 26, 2015. https://twitter.com/AnnaKendrick47/status/603273596723601408

7. Mindful Staff and Jon Kabat-Zinn, "Jon Kabat-Zinn: Defining Mindfulness". January 11, 2017. In *Mindful* magazine, Mindful Communications & Such, PBC. https://www.mindful.org/jon-kabat-zinn-defining-mindfulness/

8. S. Renee Taylor, *The Body Is Not an Apology: The Power of Radical Self-Love*, 2nd Revised Edition, Berrett-Koehler Publishers, 2021.

9. L. Rinzler, *The Buddha Walks into A Bar: A Guide to Life for a New Generation*, Shambhala Publications, 2012.

10. J. Brewer, *Unwinding Anxiety: New Science Shows How to Break the Cycles of Worry and Fear to Heal Your Mind*, Avery, 2021.

11. J. Beyer, *How To Heal: A Practical Guide To Nine Natural Therapies You Can Use To Release Your Trauma*, Jessi Beyer, 2020.

12. H. Thompson and J. Beyer, "Ep #29: Jessi Beyer: How to Heal from Trauma and Talk Openly About Mental Health (and Why Dogs Are The Best)", July 14, 2020. In *The Breathe Like A Badass Podcast*, Podcast, MP3 audio, breathelikeabadass.com/podcast

13. *Ibid.*

14. P. Ogden and J. Fisher, *Sensorimotor Psychotherapy: Interventions for Trauma and Attachment*, W.W. Norton, 2015.

15. L. Gottlieb, *Maybe You Should Talk to Someone: A therapist, her therapist, and our lives revealed*, Houghton Mifflin Harcourt, 2019.

16. A. Sweeney, B. Filson, A. Kennedy, L. Collinson et al., "A paradigm shift: relationships in trauma-informed mental health services", *JPsych Adv*, 2018;24(5):319-333, 10.1192/bja.2018.29.

17. D. A. Treleaven, *Trauma-Sensitive Mindfulness: Practices for Safe and Transformative Healing*, W.W. Norton & Company, 2018, p. xvii.

18. J. Welwood, *Toward a Psychology of Awakening: Buddhism, Psychotherapy, and the Path of Personal and Spiritual Transformation*, Shambhala Publications Inc., 2002.
19. D. Goleman and R. Davidson, *The Science of Meditation: How to Change Your Brain, Mind and Body*, Penguin, 2017.
20. S. Salzberg, *Real Love: The Art of Mindful Connection*, Bluebird, 2017.
21. K. Neff, *Self-Compassion: Stop Beating Yourself Up and Leave Insecurity Behind*, Hodder & Stoughton, 2011.

5. Meditation for Anxiety

1. S. Plath, *The Bell Jar* (50th Anniversary Edition), Faber & Faber, 2013.
2. A. Nin, *Seduction of the Minotaur: The Authoritative Edition* Swallow Press, 2014.
3. Timothy D. Wilson et al., "Just think: The challenges of the disengaged mind", *Science*, 04 Jul 2014 : 75-77, https://doi.org/10.1126/science.1250830.
4. NHS, Overview - Generalised anxiety disorder in adults, Crown copyright, 2018. https://www.nhs.uk/conditions/generalised-anxiety-disorder
5. S. McManus, et al., "Mental health and wellbeing in England: Adult psychiatric morbidity survey 2014", 2016.
6. N. Fineberg, et al., "The size, burden and cost of disorders of the brain in the UK", *Journal of Psychopharmacology*, 27(9), 2013, p.761–770.
7. A. Vahratian et al., "Symptoms of Anxiety or Depressive Disorder and Use of Mental Health Care Among Adults

During the COVID-19 Pandemic — United States",
Morbidity and Mortality Weekly Report (MMWR), 2021;
70:490–494, http://dx.doi.org/10.15585/mmwr.mm7013e2.

8. S.M. Chan, et al., "Ruminative and Catastrophizing
    Cognitive Styles Mediate the Association Between Daily
    Hassles and High Anxiety in Hong Kong Adolescents",
    Child Psychiatry Hum Dev 46, 57–66, 2015, https://doi.
    org/10.1007/s10578-014-0451-9.

9. V.A. Noël, et al., "Catastrophizing As a Predictor of
    Depressive and Anxious Symptoms in Children", *Cognitive
    Therapy and Research* vol. 36, pp. 311–320 (2012). https://
    doi.org/10.1007/s10608-011-9370-2.

10. N. Lukkahatai, at al., "Association of catastrophizing and
    fatigue: a systematic review", *Journal of Psychosomatic
    Research* vol. 74(2), 2013, https://doi:10.1016/j.
    jpsychores.2012.11.006.

11. E. Dickinson, *The Poems of Emily Dickinson*, Edited by R.W.
    Franklin, Harvard University Press, 1999.

12. T. Ferriss and D. Harris, "Ep #481: Dan Harris on
    Becoming 10% Happier, Hugging Inner Dragons, Self-
    Help for Skeptics, Training the Mind, and Much More".
    November 19, 2020. In *The Tim Ferriss Show*, The
    4-Hour, Tim Ferriss, 2007-2021. Podcast. https://tim.
    blog/2020/11/19/dan-harris-transcript

13. Timothy D. Wilson et al., "Just think: The challenges of the
    disengaged mind", *Science*, 04 Jul 2014 : 75-77, https://
    doi.org/10.1126/science.1250830.

14. B. van der Kolk, *The Body Keeps the Score: Mind, Brain
    and Body in the Transformation of Trauma*, Penguin, 2015.

15. D.A. Treleaven, *Trauma-Sensitive Mindfulness: Practices for Safe and Transformative Healing*, W.W. Norton & Company, 2018.

16. (*"l'Enfer, c'est les autres"*). J-P. Sartre and L. Abel, *No Exit, and Three Other Plays*, Vintage Books, 1989.

17. M. Williams and D. Penman, *Mindfulness: The Eight-Week Meditation Programme for a Frantic World*, Piatkus Books, 2011.

6. Working through Heartbreak and Grief

1. T. Swift, J. Antonoff, "This Is Me Trying", *Folklore*, Republic Records, 2020.

2. N. Ware, "Why we're unhappy – the expectation gap", TEDxKlagenfurt, TEDx Talks, 2014.

3. B. Feiler, *Life Is in the Transitions: Mastering Change in a Nonlinear Age*, Penguin Press, 2020.

4. E. Kubler-Ross and D. Kessler, *On Grief and Grieving: Finding the Meaning of Grief Through the Five Stages of Loss*, Reissue edition, Simon & Schuster UK, 2014.

5. D. Kessler, *Finding Meaning: The Sixth Stage of Grief*, Rider, 2019.

6. S. Berinato, "That Discomfort You're Feeling Is Grief", *Harvard Business Review*, March 23, 2020. https://hbr.org/2020/03/that-discomfort-youre-feeling-is-grief

7. *Ibid.*

8. P. Chödrön, *When Things Fall Apart: Heart Advice for Difficult Times*, HarperNonFiction, 2005.

9. S. Berinato, "That Discomfort You're Feeling Is Grief", Harvard Business Review, March 23, 2020. https://hbr. org/2020/03/that-discomfort-youre-feeling-is-grief

10. G. Garvey, C. Potter, M. Potter, P. Turner, R. Jupp, "New York Morning", *The Taking Off and Landing of Everything*, Alfred Publishing Co., Inc., 2014.

11. A. Fernandopulle and D Harris, *Insights*, Ten Percent Happier Meditation app, 10% Happier Inc., 2021.

12. L. Sheridan, *The Comparison Cure: How to be less 'them' and more you*, Orion Spring, 2019.

7. Meditation for Owning It

1. UK Small Business Statistics report, Federation of Small Businesses, 2020. https://www.fsb.org.uk/uk-small-business-statistics.html

2. L. Rosling, "64% of Britain's Workforce Wants To Set Up Their Own Business", *SME Loans*, 2019. https://smeloans. co.uk/blog/motivation-in-the-workplace-statistics

3. SBA Office of Advocacy, *2019 Small Business Profile*, 2019. https://cdn.advocacy.sba.gov/wp-content/uploads/2019/04/23142610/2019-Small-Business-Profiles-States-Territories.pdf

4. J. Williams, "How Digital Nomads are Shaping the World of Work", *The HR Director*, 2020. https://www.thehrdirector. com/features/flexible-working/how-digital-nomads-are-shaping-the-world-of-work-in-2020

5. E. Gannon, *The Multi-Hyphen Method: Work Less, Create More: How to Make Your Side Hustle Work For You*, Hodder & Stoughton, 2018.

6. The Startups Team, *Startups*, "The average entrepreneur", 2021. https://startups.co.uk/analysis/the-average-entrepreneur

7. L. Rosling, "64% of Britain's Workforce Wants To Set Up Their Own Business", *SME Loans*, 2019. https://smeloans.co.uk/blog/motivation-in-the-workplace-statistics

8. H. Gadsby, M. Parry, J. Olb, *Nanette*, Netflix, 2018.

9. B. Brown, *Braving the Wilderness: The quest for true belonging and the courage to stand alone*, Vermilion, 2017.

10. L. Sheridan, *The Comparison Cure: How to be less 'them' and more you*, Orion Spring, 2019.

11. F. Given, *Women Don't Owe You Pretty*, Cassell, 2020.

12. T. Morrison, *Song of Solomon*, Everyman, 1995.

13. B. Brown, *Daring Greatly: How the Courage to Be Vulnerable Transforms the Way We Live, Love, Parent, and Lead*, Penguin Life, 2015.

14. B. Feiler, "For The Love of Being Liked", *New York Times*, 2014. https://www.nytimes.com/2014/05/11/fashion/for-some-social-media-users-an-anxiety-from-approval-seeking.html

15. *Ibid.*

16. J. Hibberd, *The Imposter Cure: How to stop feeling like a fraud and escape the mind-trap of imposter syndrome*, Aster, 2019.

17. A. Lamott, *Bird by Bird: Some Instructions on Writing and Life*, Anchor Books, 1995.

18. C.S. Dweck, *Mindset – Updated Edition: Changing The Way You think To Fulfil Your Potential*, Robinson, 2017.

19. H. Thompson and J. Hwang, "Ep #33: Justine Hwang: How to Overcome Burnout, Self-Criticism and Your Fear

of Failure with Art and Creativity", August 11, 2020. In *The Breathe Like A Badass Podcast*, Podcast, MP3 audio, breathelikeabadass.com/podcast

20. I. Glass, *This American Life*, WBEZ Chicago, PRX The Public Radio Exchange, Podcast.

8. Mindful Productivity

1. The Mental Health Foundation, 2021. https://www.mentalhealth.org.uk/a-to-z/w/work-life-balance

2. *Ibid.*

3. US Travel Association, Project: Time Off and the GfK KnowledgePanel®, *The Work Martyr's Cautionary Tale: How the Millennial Experience Will Define America's Vacation Culture*, 2016. https://www.ustravel.org/toolkit/time-and-vacation-usage

4. M. Bernick, "The Overlooked Relation between Self-Esteem and Work." *Political Psychology* 3, no. 3/4, 1981: 211-20. Accessed June 6, 2021, https://doi.org/10.2307/3791149.

5. T. More, *Utopia 2020 Edition*, Independently published, 2020.

6. M.L. King Jr, *Where Do We Go from Here?: Chaos or Community? (King Legacy)*, Beacon Press, 2010.

7. Basic Income UK, About. https://www.basicincome.org.uk/reasons-support-basic-income

8. J.E. De Neve et al., "Does Employee Happiness have an Impact on Productivity?", Saïd Business School WP 2019-13, 2019. http://dx.doi.org/10.2139/ssrn.3470734

9. Health and Safety Executive (HSE), Work Related Stress, Anxiety or Depression Statistics in Great Britain, 2020, 2020. https://www.hse.gov.uk/statistics/causdis/stress.pdf

10. The World Health Organisation (WHO), International Statistical Classification of Diseases and Related Health Problems 10th Revision (ICD-11)-WHO, 2021. http://id.who.int/icd/entity/129180281.

11. Mayo Clinic Staff, "Job burnout: How to spot it and take action", Mayo Clinic, 2004. https://www.mayoclinic.org/healthy-lifestyle/adult-health/in-depth/burnout/art-20046642

12. M. Stevenson, "Employee Burnout Statistics You Need to Know", HR Exchange Network, 2020. https://www.hrexchangenetwork.com/employee-engagement/news/employee-burnout-statistics-you-need-to-know

13. TUC, "TUC calls for new tech to pave way to shorter working week and higher pay", 2018. https://www.tuc.org.uk/news/tuc-calls-new-tech-pave-way-shorter-working-week-and-higher-pay

14. T. Ferriss, *The 4-Hour Work Week: Escape the 9-5, Live Anywhere and Join the New Rich*, Vermilion, 2011.

15. A. Barnes with S. Jones, *The 4 Day Week: How the Flexible Work Revolution Can Increase Productivity, Profitability and Well-being, and Create a Sustainable Future*, Piatkus, 2020.

16. K. Paul, "Microsoft Japan tested a four-day work week and productivity jumped by 40%", *The Guardian*, November 4, 2019.

17. A. Cowburn, "Coronavirus: Rishi Sunak urged to consider four-day working week in response to pandemic", *The Independent*, June 20, 2020.

18. P. Jarvis, *Company of One: Why Staying Small is the Next Big Thing for Business*, Penguin, 2019.

19. D. Goleman, *Focus: The Hidden Driver of Excellence*, Bloomsbury Publishing, 2013.

20. D. Schawbel, "Daniel Goleman: Why Professionals Need Focus", *Forbes*, October 8, 2013.

21. D. Goleman and R. Davidson, *The Science of Meditation: How to Change Your Brain, Mind and Body*, Penguin, 2017.

22. A. Jha et al., "Mindfulness training modifies subsystems of attention", Cognitive, affective & behavioral neuroscience, 7(2), 109–119. https://doi.org/10.3758/cabn.7.2.109

23. M. Csikszentmihalyi, *Flow: The Psychology of Happiness*, Rider, 2002.

24. M.E. Raichle, "The restless brain", *Brain connectivity*, 1(1), 3–12., 2011. https://doi.org/10.1089/brain.2011.0019

25. K. Garrison, J. Brewer, et al., "Effortless awareness: using real time neurofeedback to investigate correlates of posterior cingulate cortex activity in meditators' self-report", *Frontiers in human neuroscience*, 7, 440, 2013. https://doi.org/10.3389/fnhum.2013.00440

26. Killingsworth, M. & Gilbert, D., (2010). "A Wandering Mind Is an Unhappy Mind", Science (New York, N.Y.). 330. 932. 10.1126/science.1192439.

27. The Pomodoro® Technique, Francesco Cirillo, https://francescocirillo.com

28. N. Antoinette and L. McKowen, "How Laura McKowen stays sober", November 30, 2020. In *Real Talk Radio*,

Podcast, MP3 audio, https://realtalkradiopodcast.com/
podcast/how-laura-mckowen-stays-sober

29. K. Brooks, "There's A Japanese Word For People Who Buy
More Books Than They Can Actually Read", *HuffPost US*,
April 23, 2014.

30. KKIT Creations LLC, *WeCroak and WeCroak Leap*, KKIT
Creations, 2020.

31. W.S. Rahula, "The Noble Eightfold Path", *Tricycle*
magazine, accessed 2021.

32. J. Kabat-Zinn, *Full Catastrophe Living, Revised Edition:
How to cope with stress, pain and illness using mindfulness
meditation*, Piatkus, 2013.

9. Meditation for Sleep

1. The Sleep Council, "New Toolkit to Help Employers Tackle
Sleep Deprivation", January 25, 2018. https://sleepcouncil.org.
uk/new-toolkit-to-help-employers-tackle-sleep-deprivation

2. Aviva, "Sleepless cities revealed as one in three adults
suffer from insomnia", October 27, 2017, https://www.aviva.
com/newsroom/news-releases/2017/10/Sleeplesscities-
revealed-as-one-in-three-adults-suffer-frominsomnia/.

3. K. Truong, "Sleep Statistics", *Sleep Foundation*, February 8,
2021.

4. J. Varney, "Is lack of sleep affecting your work?", *Public
Health Matters*, January 2018, https://publichealthmatters.
blog.gov.uk/2018/01/30/is-lack-of-sleep-affecting-your-work

5. M. Walker, *Why We Sleep: The New Science of Sleep and
Dreams*, Penguin, 2018. p. 299

6. *Ibid.* p. 164
7. *Ibid.* p. 5
8. *Ibid.* p. 316

10. Mindful Tech

1. A.F. Ward, K. Duke et al., "Brain Drain: The Mere Presence of One's Own Smartphone Reduces Available Cognitive Capacity", *Journal of the Association for Consumer Research* 2:2, 140-154, 2017.

2. H. Thompson and L. Kindred, "Ep #11: Mindful Tech, Self-Love, and Meditation For Your Real, Actual Life", June 29, 2019. In *The Breathe Like A Badass Podcast*, Podcast, MP3 audio, https://www.breathelikeabadass.com/podcast

3. J. Orlowski, D. Coombe, V Curtis, *The Social Dilemma*, Netflix, 2020.

4. Ofcom, "A decade of digital dependency", *Communications Market Report*, Ofcom, August 2, 2018.

5. D.G., "67+ Revealing Smartphone Statistics for 2021", TechJury, March 26, 2021. https://techjury.net/blog/smartphone-usage-statistics/#gref

6. J. De-Sola Gutiérrez, F. Rodríguez de Fonseca, G. Rubio, "Cell-Phone Addiction: A Review", *Frontiers in Psychiatry*, 7, 175, 2016. https://doi.org/10.3389/fpsyt.2016.00175

7. NHS, "Addiction: what is it?", *NHS UK*, April 18, 2015.

8. J. Orlowski, D. Coombe, V. Curtis, *The Social Dilemma*, Netflix, 2020.

9. J. Odell, *How To Do Nothing: Resisting the Attention Economy*, Melville House Publishing, 2019.

10. Google Trends, accessed June 6, 2021. https://trends. google.com/trends/explore?date=all&q=digital%20detox

11. M. Tanaka, T. Doksone, D. Bull, "Could phone footage put Myanmar's leaders in jail?", *BBC News*, June 3, 2021.

12. L. Rinzler, *Take Back Your Mind: Buddhist Advice for Anxious Times*, Paul Rinzler, 2020.

13. *Ibid.*

14. R. Brown, "Public Address Word of the Year 2020: Doomscrolling", *Public Address*, December 21, 2020.

11. Meditation for Body Confidence

1. D.F. Wallace, *This is Water: Some Thoughts, Delivered on a Significant Occasion, about Living a Compassionate Life*, Little Brown Book Group, 2009.

2. M.J. Crabbe, *Body Positive Power: How to stop dieting, make peace with your body and live*, Vermilion, 2017.

3. T. Mohr, *Playing Big: A practical guide for brilliant women like you*, Arrow, 2015.

4. R.L. Pearl et al., "Association between weight bias internalization and metabolic syndrome among treatment-seeking individuals with obesity", *Obesity*, 25 (2): 317, 2017. 10.1002/oby.21716

5. J. Tyrrell et al., "Height, body mass index, and socioeconomic status: mendelian randomisation study in UK Biobank", *British Medical Journal*, 352: i582, 2016. 10.1136/bmj.i582

6. J.B. Shinall, "Occupational Characteristics and the Obesity Wage Penalty", *Vanderbilt Law and Economics Research Paper* No. 16-12, *Vanderbilt Public Law Research Paper* No. 16-23, http://dx.doi.org/10.2139/ssrn.2379575

7. R. van der Zee, "Demoted or dismissed because of your weight? The reality of the size ceiling", *The Guardian*, August 30, 2017.

8. *Ibid.*

9. A. Cuddy, "Your body language may shape who you are", *TEDGlobal*, 2012.

10. S. Cain, *Quiet: The Power of Introverts in a World That Can't Stop Talking*, Penguin, 2013.

11. P. Chödrön, *When Things Fall Apart: Heart Advice for Difficult Times*, HarperNonFiction, 2005.

12. A. Walker, "Trans people twice as likely to be victims of crime in England and Wales", *Guardian*, July 17, 2020.

12. Mindful Self-care

1. H. Morillo Sarto, A. Barcelo-Soler, et al., "Efficacy of a mindful-eating programme to reduce emotional eating in patients suffering from overweight or obesity in primary care settings: a cluster-randomised trial protocol", *BMJ Open*, 9:e031327, 2019. 10.1136/bmjopen-2019-031327

2. M.J. Murphy, L.C. Mermelstein, et al., "The Benefits of Dispositional Mindfulness in Physical Health: A Longitudinal Study of Female College Students", *Journal of American College Health*, 60:5, 341-348, 2012, 10.1080/07448481.2011.629260

3. J.L. Kristeller, and R.Q. Wolever, "Mindfulness-based eating awareness training for treating binge eating disorder: the conceptual foundation", *Eating Disorders*, 19(1), 49–61, 2011. https://doi.org/10.1080/10640266.2011.533605

4. J.B. Nelson, "Mindful Eating: The Art of Presence While You Eat", *Diabetes spectrum: A publication of the American Diabetes Association*, 30(3), 171–174, 2017. https://doi.org/10.2337/ds17-0015

5. Q. Li, M. Kobayashi et al., "Effects of Forest Bathing on Cardiovascular and Metabolic Parameters in Middle-Aged Males," *Evidence-based complementary and alternative medicine: eCAM, 2016*, 2587381. https://doi.org/10.1155/2016/2587381

6. H. Thompson and K. Platt, audio interview for *The Breathe Like A Badass Podcast*, 2021. https://www.breathelikeabadass.com/podcast

7. J. Fields, *Uncertainty: Turning Fear and Doubt into Fuel for Brilliance*, Portfolio Penguin, 2012.

8. P. Braithwaite, "Please Stop Telling Me to Go For a Walk", *Self*, May 21, 2020.

9. C. Twohig-Bennett, and A. Jones, "The health benefits of the great outdoors: A systematic review and meta-analysis of greenspace exposure and health outcomes", *Environmental Research*, 166, 628–637, 2018. https://doi.org/10.1016/j.envres.2018.06.030

10. The University of East Anglia, "It's official -- spending time outside is good for you", *ScienceDaily*, July 6, 2018, www.sciencedaily.com/releases/2018/07/180706102842.htm

11. B. Mackie, *Jog On: How Running Saved My Life,* William Collins, 2018.

12. H. Murakami, *What I Talk About When I Talk About Running*, Vintage, 2009. A. Heminsley, *Running Like a Girl: Notes on Learning to Run*, Scribner Book Company, 2013. B. Gordon, *Eat, Drink, Run.: How I Got Fit Without Going Too Mad*, Headline, 2018.

13. M.S. Lee, J.P. Lee, et al., "Interaction with indoor plants may reduce psychological and physiological stress by suppressing autonomic nervous system activity in young adults: a randomized crossover study", *Journal of Physiological Anthropology*, 34(1), 21, 2015. https://doi.org/10.1186/s40101-015-0060-8

14. T. Bringslimark, T. Hartig, "Psychological Benefits of Indoor Plants in Workplaces: Putting Experimental Results into Context", *HortScience*, 42(3), 581–587, 2007. https://journals.ashs.org/hortsci/view/journals/hortsci/42/3/article-p581.xml

14. Mindfulness and Financial Wellbeing

1. Aegon, "Financial wellbeing", https://www.aegon.co.uk/workplace/employers/support-for-employers/financial-wellbeing.html

2. The University of Manchester and Alliance Manchester Business School, "Financial Wellbeing Guide", *The National Forum for Health & Wellbeing at Work*, 2020.

3. D. Kahneman and A. Deaton, "High income improves evaluation of life but not emotional well-being",

Proceedings of the National Academy of Sciences, Sep 2010, 201011492; 10.1073/pnas.1011492107

4. A. MacMillan, "6 Things You Must Know About Money and Happiness", *Time,* September 6, 2014.

5. C. Galicia, *S.A.V.E. Yourself: Develop the Financial Fitness to Spend in Alignment with your Values, not Ego,* Chelsea Garcia, 2020.

6. H. Thompson and C. Garcia, "Ep #31: Chelsea Galicia: How to Mindfully Manage Your Money and Spend In Alignment with Your Values, Not Your Ego." In *The Breathe Like A Badass Podcast,* 29 June, 2021. https://www.breathelikeabadass.com/podcast

7. H. Thompson and R. Freeman, "Ep #36: Becki Freeman: How to Transform Your Money Mindset and Take A 'Female-First' Approach to Massive Business Success." In *The Breathe Like A Badass Podcast,* September 10, 2021. https://www.breathelikeabadass.com/podcast

8. R. Howard, A. Goldsman, S. Nasar, *A Beautiful Mind,* Universal Pictures and DreamWorks Pictures, 2001.

15. Meditation for Activism and Actual Change

1. R. Purser, *McMindfulness: How Mindfulness Became the New Capitalist Spirituality,* Repeater Books, 2019.

2. *Ibid.*

3. Often attributed to Jiddu Krishnamurti, but also attributed to M. Vonnegut, *The Eden Express: A Memoir of Insanity,* Greenwood Press, 1984.

4. R. Purser, *McMindfulness: How Mindfulness Became the New Capitalist Spirituality,* Repeater Books, 2019.

5. O.M. Klimecki, et al., "Functional neural plasticity and associated changes in positive affect after compassion training", Cerebral cortex, 23(7), 1552–1561, 2013. https://doi.org/10.1093/cercor/bhs142

6. P. Condon, G. Desbordes, W.B. Miller, "Meditation Increases Compassionate Responses to Suffering", *Psychological Science*, 24(10) 2125–2127, 2013. https://doi.org/10.1177/0956797613485603

7. D. Goleman and R. Davidson, *The Science of Meditation: How to Change Your Brain, Mind and Body*, Penguin, 2017.

8. J. Stanley, *Every Body Yoga: Let Go of Fear, Get On the Mat, Love Your Body*, Workman Publishing, 2017.

9. L. Rinzler, *The Buddha Walks into A Bar: A Guide to Life for a New Generation*, Shambhala Publications, 2012.

10. Waking Up Course, *Waking Up: Guided Meditation*, Waking Up Course, LLC, 2021.

11. D. Harris and S. Harris, "Ep #306: A Meditator in the Arena", 2020. In *Ten Percent Happier with Dan Harris*, by ABC Audio. Podcast. https://www.tenpercent.com/podcast-episode/sam-harris-306

12. *Ibid.*

13. T.N. Hanh, *Peace Is Every Step: The Path of Mindfulness in Everyday Life*, Bantam Doubleday Dell Publishing, 1991.

14. T.N. Hanh, *Anger: Buddhist Wisdom for Cooling the Flames*, Rider, 2001.

15. T. Desmond, *How To Stay Human In A F*cked-Up World*, HarperOne, 2019.

16. H. Thompson and T. Desmond, "Ep #17: Tim Desmond: Meditation for Compassion, And Staying Human in

A F*cked Up World", September 9, 2020. In *The Breathe Like A Badass Podcast*, Podcast, MP3 audio, breathelikeabadass.com/podcast

17. *Ibid.*

18. D. Harris and S. Selassie, "Ep #252: You Can't Meditate This Away (Race, Rage, and the Responsibilities of Meditators)", 2020. In *Ten Percent Happier with Dan Harris*, by ABC Audio. Podcast. https://www.tenpercent.com/podcast-episode/sebene-selassie-252

Useful Resources

Contact me

To continue this conversation, please come over to say hi on Instagram or by email – I'd love to hear from you.

Instagram: @breathelikeabadass

Email: hannah@breathelikeabadass.com

To hear the full interviews of the podcasts referenced in this book, plus many more, visit: www.breathelikeabadass.com/podcast or subscribe anywhere you usually listen to podcasts by searching: "Breathe Like A Badass".

To access my free guided meditations, head to the free smartphone app Insight Timer and search for my series, "Meditation and Coffee", or head to: insighttimer.com/hannah.breathelikeabadass

For more on my one-to-one coaching, and free stuff including my Inner Critic quiz, head to: www.breathelikeabadass.com.

Recommended books

- Pema Chödrön, *When Things Fall Apart: Heart Advice for Difficult Times*, HarperNonFiction, 2005.
- Tim Desmond, *How To Stay Human In A Fucked-Up World*, HarperOne, 2019.
- Daniel Goleman and Richard Davidson, *The Science of Meditation: How to Change Your Brain, Mind and Body*, Penguin, 2017.
- Lori Gottlieb, *Maybe You Should Talk to Someone: A therapist, her therapist, and our lives revealed*, Houghton Mifflin Harcourt, 2019.
- Thich Nhat Hanh, *Peace Is Every Step: The Path of Mindfulness in Everyday Life*, Bantam Doubleday Dell Publishing, 1991.
- Dan Harris, *10% Happier: How I Tamed the Voice in My Head, Reduced Stress Without Losing My Edge, and Found Self-Help That Actually Works – A True Story*, Yellow Kite, 2017.
- Jon Kabat-Zinn, *Wherever You Go, There You Are: Mindfulness Meditation for Everyday Life, Tenth Anniversary Edition*, Piatkus, 2004.
- Adreanna Limbach, *Tea and Cake with Demons: A Buddhist Guide to Feeling Worthy*, Sounds True, 2019.
- Kristen Neff, *Self-Compassion: Stop Beating Yourself Up and Leave Insecurity Behind*, Hodder & Stoughton, 2011.
- Lodro Rinzler, *The Buddha Walks into A Bar: A Guide to Life for a New Generation*, Shambhala Publications, 2012.

- Sharon Salzberg, *Real Love: The Art of Mindful Connection*, Bluebird, 2017.
- Sharon Salzberg, *Lovingkindness: The Revolutionary Art of Happiness*, Shambhala Publications, 1995.
- David A. Treleaven, *Trauma-Sensitive Mindfulness: Practices for Safe and Transformative Healing*, W.W. Norton & Company, 2018.
- Mark Williams and Danny Penman, *Mindfulness: The Eight-Week Meditation Programme for a Frantic World*, Piatkus Books, 2011.

Recommended podcasts

- Ten Percent Happier with Dan Harris, by ABC Audio. TenPercent.com
- Real Talk Radio, by Nicole Antoinette. RealTalkRadioPodcast.com

Recommended apps

- *Headspace: Meditation & Sleep*, Headspace Inc., 2021.
- *Ten Percent Happier Meditation*, 10% Happier Inc., 2021.

About Us

Welbeck Balance publishes books dedicated to changing lives. Our mission is to deliver life-enhancing books to help improve your wellbeing so that you can live your life with greater clarity and meaning, wherever you are on life's journey. Our Trigger books are specifically devoted to opening up conversations about mental health and wellbeing.

Welbeck Balance and Trigger are part of the Welbeck Publishing Group – a globally recognized independent publisher based in London. Welbeck are renowned for our innovative ideas, production values and developing long-lasting content. Our books have been translated into over 30 languages in more than 60 countries around the world.

If you love books, then join the club and sign up to our newsletter for exclusive offers, extracts, author interviews and more information.

www.welbeckpublishing.com   **www.triggerhub.org**

🐦 welbeckpublish   🐦 Triggercalm
📷 welbeckpublish   📷 Triggercalm
📘 welbeckuk   📘 Triggercalm

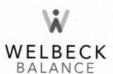

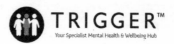